Ben Stacy Jerrik (Ed.)

Family (biology)

Ben Stacy Jerrik (Ed.)

Family (biology)

Family, Subfamily, Taxonomic, Rank, Agreement

Part Press

Imprint

Publisher:
Part Press is a trademark of
International Book Market Service Ltd., 17 Rue Meldrum, Beau Bassin, 1713-01 Mauritius
Email: info@bookmarketservice.com
Website: www.bookmarketservice.com

Published in 2012

Printed in: U.S.A., U.K., Germany. This book was not produced in Mauritius.

ISBN: 978-613-5-65753-1

Contents

Articles

Family_(biology) 1
Protein_subfamily 3
Phylum 4
Class_(biology) 10
Order_(biology) 12
Genus 14
Species 17
Domain_(biology) 29
Juglandaceae 30
Hickory 32
Taxonomic_rank 37
Taxon 46
Biological_classification 48

References

Article Sources and Contributors 56
Image Sources, Licenses and Contributors 58

Family_(biology)

In biological classification, **family** (Latin: *familia*) is

- a taxonomic rank. Other well-known ranks are life, domain, kingdom, phylum, class, order, genus, and species, with family fitting between order and genus. As for the other well-known ranks, there is the option of an immediately lower rank, indicated by the prefix *sub-*: subfamily (Latin: *subfamilia*).
- a taxonomic unit, a taxon, in that rank. In that case the plural is families (Latin *familiae*)

    Example: Walnuts and hickories belong to Juglandaceae, the walnut family.

What does and does not belong to each family is determined by a taxonomist. Similarly for the question if a particular family should be recognized at all. Often there is no exact agreement, with different taxonomists each taking a different position. There are no hard rules that a taxonomist needs to follow in describing or recognizing a family. Some taxa are accepted almost universally, while others are recognised only rarely.

The hierarchy of biological classification's eight major taxonomic ranks, which is an example of definition by genus and differentia. An order contains one or more families. Intermediate minor rankings are not shown.

History

The taxonomic term *familia* was first used by French botanist Pierre Magnol in his *Prodromus historiae generalis plantarum, in quo familiae plantarum per tabulas disponuntur* (1689) where he called the seventy-six groups of plants he recognised in his tables families (*familiae*). The concept of rank at that time was not yet settled, and in the preface to the *Prodromus* Magnol spoke of uniting his families into larger *genera*, which is far from how the term is used today.

Carolus Linnaeus used the word *familia* in his *Philosophia botanica* (1751) to denote major groups of plants: trees, herbs, ferns, palms, and so on. He used this term only in the morphological section of the book, discussing the vegetative and generative organs of plants. Subsequently, in French botanical publications, from Michel Adanson's *Familles naturelles des plantes* (1763) and until the end of the 19th century, the word *famille* was used as a French equivalent of the Latin *ordo* (or *ordo naturalis*). In nineteenth century works such as the *Prodromus* of Augustin Pyramus de Candolle and the *Genera Plantarum* of George Bentham and Joseph Dalton Hooker this word *ordo* was used for what now is given the rank of family.

In zoology, the family as a rank intermediate between order and genus was introduced by Pierre André Latreille in his *Précis des caractères génériques des insectes, disposés dans un ordre naturel* (1796). He used families (some of them not named) in some but not in all his orders of "insects" (which then included all arthropods).

Uses

Families can be used for evolutionary, palaeontological and generic studies because they are more stable than lower taxonomic levels such as genera and species.[1] [2]

See also

- Systematics, the study of the diversity of life
- Cladistics, the classification of organisms by their order of branching in an evolutionary tree
- Phylogenetics, the study of evolutionary relatedness among various groups of organisms
- Taxonomy
- Virus classification
- List of Anuran families
- List of Testudines families
- List of fish families
- List of families of spiders

Compare:

- family
- protein family
- gene family

References

[1] Sarda Sahney, Michael J. Benton & Paul A. Ferry (2010). "Links between global taxonomic diversity, ecological diversity and the expansion of vertebrates on land" (http://rsbl.royalsocietypublishing.org/content/6/4/544.full.pdf+html) (PDF). *Biology Letters* **6** (4): 544–547. doi:10.1098/rsbl.2009.1024. PMC 2936204. PMID 20106856. .

[2] Sarda Sahney & Michael J. Benton (2008). "Recovery from the most profound mass extinction of all time" (http://journals.royalsociety.org/content/qq5un1810k7605h5/fulltext.pdf) (PDF). *Proceedings of the Royal Society B: Biological Sciences* **275** (1636): 759–765. doi:10.1098/rspb.2007.1370. PMC 2596898. PMID 18198148. .

Protein_subfamily

Protein subfamily is a level of protein classification, especially protein 3D structures. It is under protein family. Protein family in SCOP (Structural Classification of Proteins) means the members are all related evolutionarily and they share very similar structures with functional similarities. Protein subfamily is when the family members share the same interaction interfaces and interaction partners. This more strict criterion forces that all the subfamily members have to share functionally related.

External links

- SCOP DB at Cambridge UK [1]
- CATH protein structure DB [2]
- ProteinSubfamily wiki portal [3]

References

[1] http://www.scop.mrc-lmb.cam.ac.uk/scop
[2] http://cathdb.info
[3] http://proteinsubfamily.org

Phylum

In biology, a **phylum** (English pronunciation: /ˈfaɪləm/; plural: **phyla**)[1] is a taxonomic rank below kingdom and above class. "Phylum" is equivalent to the botanical term **division**.[2] The kingdom Animalia contains approximately 35 phyla; the kingdom Plantae contains 12 divisions. Current research in phylogenetics is uncovering the relationships between phyla, which are contained in larger clades, like Ecdysozoa and Embryophyta.

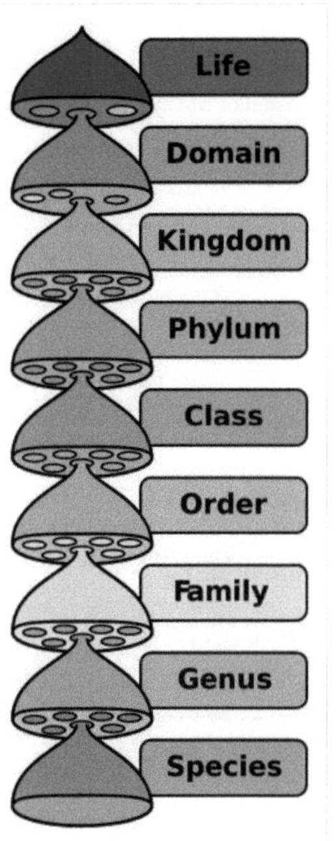

The hierarchy of biological classification's eight major taxonomic ranks, which is an example of definition by genus and differentia. A kingdom contains one or more phyla. Intermediate minor rankings are not shown.

General description and familiar examples

Informally, phyla can be thought of as grouping organisms based on general specialization of body plan,[3] At the most basic level, a phylum can be defined in two ways: as a group of organisms with a certain degree of morphological or developmental similarity (the phenetic definition), or a group of organisms with a certain degree of evolutionary relatedness (the phylogenetic definition).[4] Attempting to define a level of the Linnean hierarchy without referring to (evolutionary) relatedness is an unsatisfactory approach, but the phenetic definition is more useful when addressing questions of a morphological nature—such as how successful different body plans were.

Definition based on genetic relation

The largest objective measure in the above definitions is the "certain degree"—how unrelated do organisms need to be to be members of different phyla? The minimal requirement is that all organisms in a phylum should be related closely enough for them to be clearly more closely related to one another than to any other group.[4] However, even this is problematic, as the requirement depends on our current knowledge about organisms' relationships: As more data becomes available, particularly from molecular studies, we are better able to judge the relationships between groups. So phyla can be merged or split if it becomes apparent that they are related to one another or not. For example, the bearded worms were described as a new phylum (the Pogonophora) when described in 1914, but molecular work almost a century later found them closely related to annelids and merged the phyla, so that the bearded worms are now an annelid family.[5] Likewise, the highly parasitic phylum Mesozoa was divided into two phyla Orthonectida and Rhombozoa, when it was discovered the Orthonectida are deuterostomes and the Rhombozoa protostomes.[6]

This changeability of phyla has led some biologists to call for the concept of a phylum to be abandoned in favour of cladistics, a method in which plan" based definition of a phylum has been proposed by paleontologists Graham Budd and Sören Jensen. The definition was posited by paleontologists off-shoots that diverged from a phylum's history before the characters that define the modern phylum were all acquired!

Definition based on body plan

By Budd and Jensen's definition, phyla are defined by a set of characters shared by all their living representatives. This has a couple of small problems—for instance, characters common to most members of a phylum may be secondarily lost by some members. It is also defined based on an arbitrary point of time (the present). However, as it is character based, it is easy to apply to the fossil record. A more major problem is that it relies on an objective decision of which group of organisms should be considered a phylum.

Its utility is that it makes it easy to classify extinct organisms as "stem groups" to the phyla with which they bear the most resemblance, based only on the taxonomically important similarities.[4] However, proving that a fossil belongs to the crown group of a phylum is difficult, as it must display a character unique to a sub-set of the crown group.[4] aspects of the "body plan" of the phylum without all the characters necessary to fall within it. This weakens the idea that each of the phyla represents a distinct body plan.[7]

Based upon this definition, which some say is unreasonably affected by the chance survival of rare groups, which vastly increase the size of phyla, representatives of many modern phyla did not appear until long *after* the Cambrian.[8]

Lists

Animal phyla

Phylum	Meaning	Common name	Distinguishing characteristic	Species described
Acanthocephala	Thorny headed worms	Thorny-headed worms	Reversible spiny proboscis	approx. 756
Acoelomorpha	Without gut	Acoels	No mouth or alimentary canal (alimentary canal = digestive tract in digestive system)	
Annelida	Little ring	Segmented worms	Multiple circular segment	17000+ extant
Arthropoda	Jointed foot	Arthropods	Chitin exoskeleton	1134000+
Brachiopoda	Arm foot	Lamp shells	Lophophore and pedicle	300-500 extant
Bryozoa	Moss animals	Moss animals, sea mats	Lophophore, no pedicle, ciliated tentacles	5000 extant
Chaetognatha	Longhair jaw	Arrow worms	Chitinous spines either side of head, fins	approx. 100 extant
Chordata	Cord	Chordates	Hollow dorsal nerve cord, notochord, pharyngeal slits, endostyle, post-anal tail	approx. 100000+
Cnidaria	Stinging nettle	Coelenterates	Nematocysts (stinging cells)	approx. 11000
Ctenophora	Comb bearer	Comb jellies	Eight "comb rows" of fused cilia	approx. 100 extant
Cycliophora	Wheel carrying	Symbion	Circular mouth surrounded by small cilia	3+
Echinodermata	Spiny skin	Echinoderms	Fivefold radial symmetry in living forms, mesodermal calcified spines	approx. 7000 extant; approx. 13,000 extinct
Entoprocta	Inside anus	Goblet worm	Anus inside ring of cilia	approx. 150
Gastrotricha	Hair stomach	Meiofauna	Two terminal adhesive tubes	approx. 690
Gnathostomulida	Jaw orifice	Jaw worms		approx. 100
Hemichordata	Half cord	Acorn worms, pterobranchs	Stomochord in collar, pharyngeal slits	approx. 100 extant
Kinorhyncha	Motion snout	Mud dragons	Eleven segments, each with a dorsal plate	approx. 150
Loricifera	Corset bearer	Brush heads	Umbrella-like scales at each end	approx. 122

Micrognathozoa	Tiny jaw animals	—	Accordion like extensible thorax	1
Mollusca	Soft	Mollusks / molluscs	Muscular foot and mantle round shell	112000[9]
Nematoda	Thread like	Round worms	Round cross section, keratin cuticle	80000–1,000,000
Nematomorpha	Thread form	Horsehair worms		approx. 320
Nemertea	A sea nymph	Ribbon worms		approx. 1200
Onychophora	Claw bearer	Velvet worms	Legs tipped by chitinous claws	approx. 200 extant
Orthonectida	Straight swim		Single layer of ciliated cells surrounding a mass of sex cells	approx. 20
Phoronida	Zeus's mistress	Horseshoe worms	U-shaped gut	20
Placozoa	Plate animals			1
Platyhelminthes	Flat worms	Flat worms		approx. 25000[10]
Porifera*	Pore bearer	Sponges	Perforated interior wall	5000+ extant
Priapulida	Little Priapus			16
Rhombozoa	Lozenge animal	—	Single axial cell surrounded by ciliated cells	75
Rotifera	Wheel bearer	Rotifers	Anterior crown of cilia	approx. 2000
Sipuncula	Small tube	Peanut worms	Mouth surrounded by invertible tentacles	144–320
Tardigrada	Slow step	Water bears	Four segmented body and head	1000+
Xenoturbellida	Strange flatworm	—	Ciliated deuterostome	2
Total: 35				**2,000,000-**

Protostome	Bilateria
Deuterostome	
Basal/disputed	
Other	

Groups formerly ranked as phyla

Name as phylum	Common name	Current consensus
Aschelminthes	Pseudocoelomates	Divided into several pseudocoelomate phyla.
Craniata	—	Subgroup of phylum Chordata; perhaps synonymous with Vertebrata.
Cephalochordata	Lancelets	Subphylum of phylum Chordata.
Cephalorhyncha	—	Superphylum Scalidophora.
Echiura	Spoon worms	Class of phylum Annelida.
Enterepneusta	Acorn worms	Class of phylum Hemichordata.
Gephyra	Peanut worms and spoon worms	Divided into phyla Sipuncula and Echiura.
Mesozoa	Mesozoans	Divided into phyla Orthonectida and Rhombozoa.
Myxozoa		Severely modified Cnidarians.
Pentastomida	Tongue worms	Subclass of Maxillopoda of phylum Arthropoda.

Pogonophora	Beard worms	Part of family Siboglinidae of phylum Annelida.
Pterobranchia	—	Class of phylum Hemichordata.
Symplasma	Glass sponges	Class Hexactinellida of phylum Porifera.
Urochordata	Tunicates	Subphylum of phylum Chordata.
Vestimentifera	Vent worms	Part of family Siboglinidae of phylum Annelida.

Plant divisions

Division	**Meaning**	**Common name**	**Distinguishing characteristics**
Anthocerotophyta	Flower-horn plants	Hornworts	Horn-shaped sporophytes, no vascular system
Bryophyta	Moss plants	Mosses	Persistent unbranched sporophytes, no vascular system
Marchantiophyta	*Marchantia* plants	Liverworts	Ephemeral unbranched sporophytes, no vascular system
Lycopodiophyta	Wolf foot plants	Clubmosses & Spikemosses	Microphyll leaves, vascular system
Pteridophyta	Fern plants	Ferns & Horsetails	Prothallus gametophytes, vascular system
Pteridospermatophyta	Fern with seeds plant	Seed ferns	Only known from fossils, mostly Devonian, ranking in dispute[11]
Coniferophyta	Sap/pitch plants	Conifers	Cones containing seeds and wood composed of tracheids
Cycadophyta	Palm plants	Cycads	Seeds, crown of compound leaves
Ginkgophyta	Ginkgo plants	Ginkgo, Maidenhair	Seeds not protected by fruit (single species)
Gnetophyta		Gnetophytes	Seeds and woody vascular system with vessels
Anthophyta (or Magnoliophyta)	Flower plant	Flowering plants	Flowers and fruit, vascular system with vessels

Fungal divisions

Phylum	**Meaning**	**Common name**	**Distinguishing characteristics**
Chytridiomycota	Little pot mushroom	Chytrids	Cellulose in cell walls, flagellated gametes
Deuteromycota	Second mushroom	Imperfect fungi	Unclassified fungi; only asexual reproduction observed
Zygomycota	Yolk mushroom	Zygomycetes	Blend gametangia to form a zygosporangium
Glomeromycota	Ball mushroom	None	Form arbuscular mycorrhizae with plants
Ascomycota	Bag/Wineskin Mushroom	Sac fungi	Produce spores in an 'ascus'
Basidiomycota	Basidium Mushroom	Club Fungi	Produce spores from a 'basidium'

Bacterial Phyla/Divisions

Currently there are 29 phyla accepted by LPSN[12]

1. Acidobacteria, phenotipically diverse and mostly uncultured
2. Actinobacteria, High-G+C Gram positive species
3. Aquificae, only 14 thermophilic genera, deep branching
4. Bacteroidetes
5. Caldiserica, formerly candidate division OP5, *Caldisericum exile* is the sole representative
6. Chlamydiae, only 6 genera
7. Chlorobi, only 7 genera
8. Chloroflexi,
9. Chrysiogenetes, only 3 genera (*Chrysiogenes arsenatis*, *Desulfurispira natronophila*, *Desulfurispirillum alkaliphilum*)
10. Cyanobacteria, also known as the blue-green algae
11. Deferribacteres
12. Deinococcus-Thermus, *Deinococcus radiodurans* and *Thermus aquaticus* are "commonly known" species of this phyla
13. Dictyoglomi
14. Elusimicrobia, formerly candidate division Thermite Group 1
15. Fibrobacteres
16. Firmicutes, Low-G+C Gram positive species, such as the spore-formers Bacilli (aerobic) and Clostridia (anaerobic)
17. Fusobacteria
18. Gemmatimonadetes
19. Lentisphaerae, formerly clade VadinBE97
20. Nitrospira
21. Planctomycetes ANo ito?
22. Proteobacteria, the most known phyla, containing species such as *Escherichia coli* or *Pseudomonas aeruginosa*
23. Spirochaetes, species include *Borrelia burgdorferi*, which causes Lyme disease
24. Synergistetes
25. Tenericutes, alternatively class Mollicutes in phylum Firmicutes (notable genus: *Mycoplasma*)
26. Thermodesulfobacteria
27. Thermomicrobia
28. Thermotogae, deep branching
29. Verrucomicrobia

Archaeal Phyla/Division

1. Crenarchaeota, Second most common archaeal phylum
2. Euryarchaeota, most common archaeal phylum
3. Korarchaeota
4. Nanoarchaeota, ultra-small symbiotes
5. Thaumarchaeota

See also

- Cladistics
- Phylogenetics
- Systematics
- Taxonomy

Notes

[1] The term was coined by Georges Cuvier from Greek φῦλον *phylon*, "race, stock," related to φυλή *phyle*, "tribe, clan."

[2] "Life sciences" (http://dictionary.reference.com/browse/phylum). *The American Heritage New Dictionary of Cultural Literacy* (third ed.). Houghton Mifflin Company. 2005. . Retrieved 2008-10-04. "Phyla in the plant kingdom are frequently called divisions."

[3] Valentine, James W. (2004). *On the Origin of Phyla*. Chicago: University Of Chicago Press. pp. 7. ISBN 0226845486. "Classifications of organisms in hierarchical systems were in use by the seventeenth and eighteenth centuries. Usually organisms were grouped according to their what? morphological similarities as perceived by those early workers, and those groups were then grouped according to their similarities, and so on, to form a hierarchy."

[4] Budd, G.E.; Jensen, S. (2000). "A critical reappraisal of the fossil record of the bilaterian phyla" (http://www.journals.cambridge.org/abstract_S000632310000548X). *Biological Reviews* **75** (2): 253–295. doi:10.1017/S000632310000548X. PMID 10881389. . Retrieved 2007-05-26.

[5] Rouse G.W. (2001). "A cladistic analysis of Siboglinidae Caullery, 1914 (Polychaeta, Annelida): formerly the phyla Pogonophora and Vestimentifera". *Zoological Journal of the Linnean Society* **132** (1): 55–80. doi:10.1006/zjls.2000.0263.

[6] Pawlowski J, Montoya-Burgos JI, Fahrni JF, Wüest J, Zaninetti L (October 1996). "Origin of the Mesozoa inferred from 18S rRNA gene sequences" (http://mbe.oxfordjournals.org/cgi/pmidlookup?view=long&pmid=8865666). *Mol. Biol. Evol.* **13** (8): 1128–32. PMID 8865666. .

[7] Budd, G.E. (1998). "Arthropod body-plan evolution in the Cambrian with an example from anomalocaridid muscle" (http://www.blackwell-synergy.com/doi/abs/10.1111/j.1502-3931.1998.tb00508.x). *Lethaia* (Blackwell Synergy) **31** (3): 197–210. doi:10.1111/j.1502-3931.1998.tb00508.x. .

[8] Briggs, D. E. G; Fortey, R. A (2005). "Wonderful strife: systematics, stem groups, and the phylogenetic signal of the Cambrian radiation". *Paleobiology* **31** (2 (Suppl)): 94–112. doi:10.1666/0094-8373(2005)031[0094:WSSSGA]2.0.CO;2.

[9] Feldkamp, S. (2002) *Modern Biology*. Holt, Rinehart, and Winston, USA. (pp. 725)

[10] Species Register. "Flatworms — Phylum Platyhelminthes" (http://www.woodbridge.tased.edu.au/mdc/Species Register/phylum_platyhelminthes.htm). Marine Discovery Centres. . Retrieved 2007-04-09.

[11] ""Kingdom Plantae Tree of Life"" (http://www.fossilmuseum.net/Tree_of_Life/KingdomPlantae.htm). .

[12] J.P. Euzéby. "List of Prokaryotic names with Standing in Nomenclature: Phyla" (http://www.bacterio.cict.fr/classifphyla.html). . Retrieved 30 December 2010.

References

External links

- Are phyla "real"? Is there really a well-defined "number of animal phyla" extant and in the fossil record? (http://www.pandasthumb.org/archives/2005/04/down_with_phyla_1.html)
- Major Phyla Of Animals (http://waynesword.palomar.edu/trnov01.htm)

Class_(biology)

In biological classification, **class** (Latin: *classis*) is

- a taxonomic rank. Other well-known ranks are life, domain, kingdom, phylum, order, family, genus, and species, with class fitting between phylum and order. As for the other well-known ranks, there is the option of an immediately lower rank, indicated by the prefix *sub-*: subclass (Latin: *subclassis*).
- a taxonomic unit, a taxon, in that rank. In that case the plural is classes (Latin *classes*)

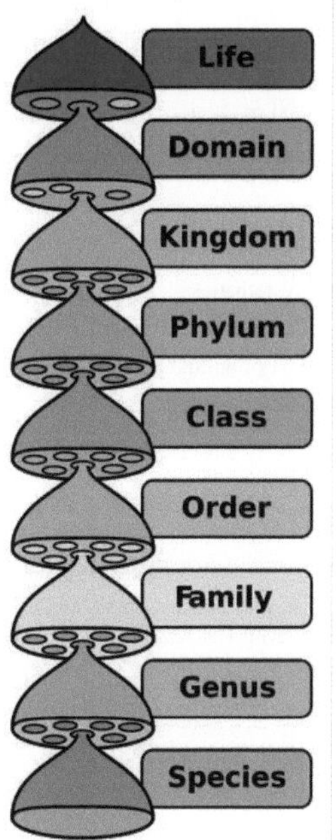

The hierarchy of biological classification's eight major taxonomic ranks, which is an example of definition by genus and differentia. Intermediate minor rankings are not shown.

The composition of each class is determined by a taxonomist. Often there is no exact agreement, with different taxonomists taking different positions. There are no hard rules that a taxonomist needs to follow in describing a class, but for well-known animals there is likely to be consensus. For example, dogs are usually assigned to the phylum Chordata (animals with notochords); in the class Mammalia; in the order Carnivora.

Hierarchy of ranks

For some clades, a number of additional classifications are used. The different classes are used relatively rarely.

Name	Meaning of prefix	Example 1	Example 2	Example 3[1]
Superclass	super: above	Tetrapoda		
Class		Mammalia	Maxillopoda	Sauropsida
Subclass	sub: under		Thecostraca	Avialae
Infraclass	infra: below		Cirripedia	Aves
Parvclass	parvus: small, unimportant			Neornithes

History of the concept

The class as a distinct rank of biological classification having its own distinctive name (and not just called a *top-level genus (genus summum)* was first introduced by the French botanist Joseph Pitton de Tournefort in his classification of plants (it appeared in his 1694 *Eléments de botanique*). Carolus Linnaeus was the first to use it consistently, in dividing of all three of his kingdoms of Nature (minerals, plants, and animals) in his *Systema Naturae* (1735, 1st ed.).[2] Since then the class was considered the highest level of the taxonomic hierarchy until the *embranchements*, now called phyla, and divisions were introduced in the nineteenth century.

See also

- Systematics
- Cladistics
- List of animal classes
- Phylogenetics
- Taxonomy

References

[1] Classification according to Systema Naturae 2000, which conflicts with Wikipedia's classification. "The Taxonomicon: Neornithes" (http://taxonomicon.taxonomy.nl/TaxonTree.aspx?id=1014031). . Retrieved 3 December 2010.
[2] Mayr E. (1982). *The Growth of Biological Thought*. Cambridge: The Belknap Press of Harvard University Press. ISBN 0-674-36446-5

Order_(biology)

In scientific classification used in biology, the **order** (Latin: *ordo*) is

1. a taxonomic rank used in the classification of organisms. Other well-known ranks are life, domain, kingdom, phylum, class, family, genus, and species, with order fitting in between class and family. An immediately higher rank, **superorder**, may be added directly above order, while **suborder** would be a lower rank.
2. a taxonomic unit, a taxon, in that rank. In that case the plural is orders (Latin *ordines*).

> *Example*: Walnuts and hickories belong to the family Juglandaceae (or walnut family), which is placed in the order Fagales.

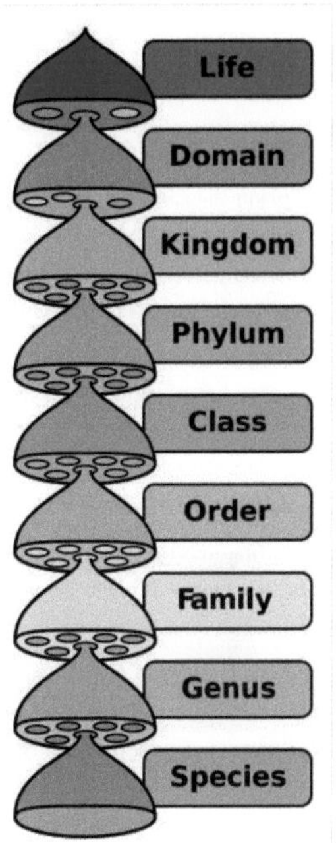

The hierarchy of biological classification's eight major taxonomic ranks, which is an example of definition by genus and differentia. A class contains one or more orders. Intermediate minor rankings are not shown.

What does and does not belong to each order is determined by a taxonomist. Similarly for the question if a particular order should be recognized at all. Often there is no exact agreement, with different taxonomists each taking a different position. There are no hard rules that a taxonomist needs to follow in describing or recognizing an order. Some taxa are accepted almost universally, while others are recognised only rarely.

For some groups of organisms, consistent suffixes are used to denote that the rank is an order. The Latin suffix *-(i)formes* meaning "having the form of" is used for the scientific name of orders of birds and fishes, but not for those of mammals and invertebrates. The suffix *-ales* is for the name of orders of vascular plants.

Hierarchy of ranks

For some clades, a number of additional classifications are used.

Name	Meaning of prefix	Example
Magnorder	magnus: large, great, important	Epitheria
Superorder	super: above	Euarchontoglires
Order		Primates
Suborder	sub: under	Haplorrhini
Infraorder	infra: below	Simiiformes
Parvorder	parvus: small, unimportant	Catarrhini

In their 1997 classification of mammals, McKenna and Bell used two extra levels between Superorder and Order: "Grandorder" and "Mirorder".[1]

History of the concept

The order as a distinct rank of biological classification having its own distinctive name (and not just called a *higher genus (genus summum))* was first introduced by a German botanist Augustus Quirinus Rivinus in his classification of plants (appeared in a series of treatises in the 1690s). Carolus Linnaeus was the first to apply it consistently to the division of all three kingdoms of nature (minerals, plants, and animals) in his *Systema Naturae* (1735, 1st. Ed.).

Botany

For plants the Linnaean orders, in the *Systema Naturae* and the *Species Plantarum*, were strictly artificial, introduced to subdivide the artificial classes into more comprehensible smaller groups. When the word *ordo* was first consistently used for natural units of plants, in nineteenth century works such as the *Prodromus* of de Candolle and the *Genera Plantarum* of Bentham & Hooker, it indicated taxa that are now given the rank of family (see *ordo naturalis*).

In French botanical publications, from Michel Adanson's *Familles naturelles des plantes* (1763) and until the end of the 19th century, the word *famille* (plural: *familles*) was used as a French equivalent for this Latin *ordo*. This equivalence was explicitly stated in the Alphonse De Candolle's *Lois de la nomenclature botanique* (1868), the precursor of the currently used *International Code of Botanical Nomenclature*.

In the first international *Rules* of botanical nomenclature of 1906 the word family (*familia*) was assigned to the rank indicated by the French "famille", while order (*ordo*) was reserved for a higher rank, for what in the nineteenth century had often been named a *cohors* (plural *cohortes*).

Some of the plant families still retain the names of Linnaean "natural orders" or even the names of pre-Linnaean natural groups recognised by Linnaeus as orders in his natural classification (e.g. *Palmae* or *Labiatae*). Such names are known as descriptive family names.

Zoology

In zoology, the Linnaean orders were used more consistently. That is, the orders in the zoology part of the *Systema Naturae* refer to natural groups. Some of his ordinal names are still in use (e.g. Lepidoptera for the order of moths and butterflies, or Diptera for the order of flies, mosquitoes, midges, and gnats).

See also

- Cladistics
- Phylogenetics
- Rank (botany)
- Rank (zoology)
- Biological classification
- Systematics
- Taxonomy
- Virus classification

References

[1] McKenna, M.C. & Bell, S.G. (1997), *Classification of Mammals*, New York: Columbia University Press, ISBN 978-0-231-11013-6

Genus

In biology, a **genus** (plural: **genera**) is a low-level taxonomic rank used in the biological classification of living and fossil organisms, which is an example of definition by genus and differentia. Genera and higher taxonomic levels such as families are used in biodiversity studies, particularly in fossil studies since species cannot always be confidently identified and genera and families typically have longer stratigraphic ranges than species.[1]

The term comes from Latin genus "descent, family, type, gender",[2] cognate with Greek: *γένος* – *genos*, "race, stock, kin".[3]

The composition of a genus is determined by a taxonomist. The standards for genus classification are not strictly codified so different authorities often produce different classifications for genera. In the hierarchy of the binomial classification system, genus comes above species and below family.

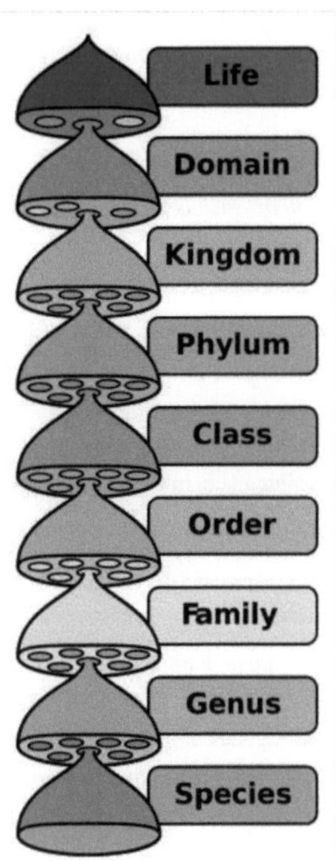

The hierarchy of biological classification's eight major taxonomic ranks, which is an example of definition by genus and differentia. A family contains one or more genera. Intermediate minor rankings are not shown.

Generic name

The scientific name of a genus may be called the **generic name** or **generic epithet**: it is always capitalized. It plays a pivotal role in binomial nomenclature, the system of biological nomenclature.

Binomial nomenclature

The rules for scientific names (Binomial Nomenclature) are laid down in the Nomenclature Codes; depending on the kind of organism and the Kingdom it belongs to, a different Code may apply, with different rules, laid down in a different terminology. The advantages of scientific over common names are that they are accepted by speakers of all languages, and that each species has only one name. This reduces the confusion that may arise from the use of a common name to designate different things in different places (example elk), or from the existence of several common names for a single species.

It is possible for a genus to be assigned to a kingdom governed by one particular Nomenclature Code by one taxonomist, while other taxonomists assign it to a kingdom governed by a different Code, but this is the exception, not the rule.

Pivotal in binomial nomenclature

The generic name is a component of the names of taxa of lower rank. For example, *Canis lupus* is the scientific name of the Gray wolf, a species, with *Canis* the generic name for the dog and its close relatives, and with *lupus* particular (specific) for the wolf (*lupus* is written in lower case). Similarly, *Canis lupus familiaris* is the scientific name for the domestic dog.

Taxonomic units in higher ranks often have a name that is based on a generic name, such as the family name Canidae, which is based on *Canis*. However, not all names in higher ranks are necessarily based on the name of a genus: for example, Carnivora is the name for the order to which the dog belongs.

Identical names used for different genera

A genus in one kingdom is allowed to bear a scientific name that is in use as a generic name (or the name of a taxon in another rank) in a kingdom that is governed by a different nomenclature code. Although this is discouraged by both the International Code of Zoological Nomenclature and the International Code of Botanical Nomenclature, there are some five thousand such names in use in more than one kingdom. For instance, *Anura* is the name of the order of frogs but also is the name of a genus of plants (although not current: it is a synonym); *Aotus* is the genus of golden peas and night monkeys; *Oenanthe* is the genus of wheatears and water dropworts, *Prunella* is the genus of accentors and self-heal, and *Proboscidea* is the order of elephants and the genus of devil's claws.

Within the same kingdom one generic name can apply to only one genus. This explains why the platypus genus is named *Ornithorhynchus*—George Shaw named it *Platypus* in 1799, but the name *Platypus* had already been given to a group of ambrosia beetles by Johann Friedrich Wilhelm Herbst in 1793. Names with the same form but applying to different taxa are called homonyms. Since beetles and platypuses are both members of the kingdom Animalia, the name *Platypus* could not be used for both. Johann Friedrich Blumenbach published the replacement name *Ornithorhynchus* in 1800.

Types and genera

Because of the rules of scientific naming, or "binomial nomenclature", each genus should have a designated type, although in practice there is a backlog of older names that may not yet have a type. In zoology this is the type species; the generic name is permanently associated with the type specimen of its type species. Should this specimen turn out to be assignable to another genus, the generic name linked to it becomes a junior synonym, and the remaining taxa in the former genus need to be reassessed.

See scientific classification and nomenclature codes for more details of this system. Also see type genus.

Guidelines

There are no hard and fast rules that a taxonomist has to follow in deciding what does and what does not belong in a particular genus. This does not mean that there is no common ground among taxonomists in what constitutes a "good" genus. For instance, some rules-of-thumb for delimiting a genus are outlined in Gill.[4] According to these, a genus should fulfill three criteria to be descriptively useful:

1. monophyly – all descendants of an ancestral taxon are grouped together;
2. reasonable compactness – a genus should not be expanded needlessly; and
3. distinctness – in regards of evolutionarily relevant criteria, i.e. ecology, morphology, or biogeography; note that DNA sequences are a *consequence* rather than a *condition* of diverging evolutionary lineages except in cases where they directly inhibit gene flow (e.g. postzygotic barriers).

Nomenclature

...difficulties occurring in generic nomenclature: similar cases abound, and become complicated by the different views taken of the matter by the various taxonomists.

Prof. C. S. Rafinesque. 1836[5]

None of the nomenclature codes require such criteria for defining a genus, because these are concerned with the nomenclature rules, not with taxonomy. These regulate formal nomenclature, aiming for universal and stable scientific names.

See also

- List of the largest genera of flowering plants

References

[1] Sahney, S., Benton, M.J. and Ferry, P.A. (2010). "Links between global taxonomic diversity, ecological diversity and the expansion of vertebrates on land" (http://rsbl.royalsocietypublishing.org/content/6/4/544.full.pdf+html) (PDF). *Biology Letters* **6** (4): 544–547. doi:10.1098/rsbl.2009.1024. PMC 2936204. PMID 20106856. .

[2] Merriam Webster Dictionary (http://www.merriam-webster.com/dictionary/genus)

[3] Genos (http://www.perseus.tufts.edu/cgi-bin/ptext?doc=Perseus:text:1999.04.0057:entry=#21921), Henry George Liddell, Robert Scott, 'A Greek-English Lexicon, *at Perseus*

[4] Gill, F. B., B. Slikas, and F. H. Sheldon. "Phylogeny of titmice (Paridae): II. Species relationships based on sequences of the mitochondrial cytochrome-b gene." Auk 122(1): 121-143, 2005. (Google Scholar) (http://scholar.google.com/scholar?cluster=16219444564703958615&hl=en)

[5] Rafinesque, Prof. C. S. (1836). "Generic Rules" (http://www.us.archive.org/GnuBook/?id=floratellurianaOOrafi#99). *Flora telluriana Pars Prima First Part of the Synoptical Flora Telluriana, Centuries I, II, III, IV. With new Natural Classes, Orders and families: containing the 2000 New or revised Genera and Species of Trees, Palms, Shrubs, Vines, Plants, Lilies, Grasses, Ferns, Algas, Fungi, & c. from North and South America, Polynesia, Australia, Asia Europe and Africa, omitted or mistaken by the authors, that were observed or ascertained, described or revised, collected or figured, between 1796 and 1836.* (http://www.us.archive.org/GnuBook/?id=floratellurianaOOrafi#13). **1**. Philadelphia: H. Probasco. . Retrieved 2009-04-02. "...difficulties occurring in generic nomenclature: similar cases abound, and become complicated by the different views taken of the matter by the various botanists."

External links

- Nomenclator Zoologicus (http://uio.mbl.edu/NomenclatorZoologicus/): Index of all genus and subgenus names in zoological nomenclature from 1758 to 2004.
- Fauna Europaea Database for Taxonomy (http://www.faunaeur.org/full_results.php?id=193482)

Species

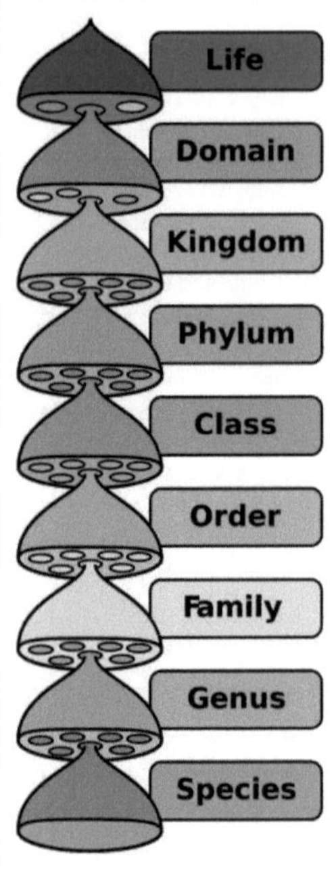

The hierarchy of biological classification's eight major taxonomic ranks, which is an example of definition by genus and differentia. A genus contains one or more species. Intermediate minor rankings are not shown.

In biology, a **species** is one of the basic units of biological classification and a taxonomic rank. A species is often defined as a group of organisms capable of interbreeding and producing fertile offspring. While in many cases this definition is adequate, more precise or differing measures are often used, such as similarity of DNA, morphology or ecological niche. Presence of specific locally adapted traits may further subdivide species into "infraspecific taxa" such as subspecies (and in botany other taxa are used, such as varieties, subvarieties, and formae).

Species that are believed to have the same ancestors are grouped together, and this group is called a genus. A species will be placed in only one genus (although taxonomic opinion might change). Similarity is best checked by the similarity of their DNA, but for practical reasons, other properties are used. All species are given a two-part name, a "binomial name". The first part of a binomial name is the generic name, the genus of the species. The second part is either called the specific name (a term used only in zoology) or the specific epithet (the term used in botany, which can also be used in zoology). For example, *Boa constrictor* is one of four species of the *Boa* genus. The first part of the name is capitalized, and the second part has a lower case. The binomial name is written in italics.

A usable definition of the word "species" and reliable methods of identifying particular species are essential for stating and testing biological theories and for measuring biodiversity, though other taxonomic levels such as families may be considered in broad-scale studies.[1] Extinct species known only from fossils are generally difficult to assign precise taxonomic rankings, which is why higher taxonomic levels such as families are often used for fossil-based studies.[1] [2]

The total number of non-bacterial species in the world has been estimated at 8.7 million,[3] with previous estimates ranging from two million to 100 million.[4]

Biologists' working definition

A usable definition of the word "species" and reliable methods of identifying particular species is essential for stating and testing biological theories and for measuring biodiversity. Traditionally, multiple examples of a proposed species must be studied for unifying characters before it can be regarded as a species. It is generally difficult to give precise taxonomic rankings to extinct species known only from fossils.

Some biologists may view species as statistical phenomena, as opposed to the traditional idea, with a species seen as a class of organisms. In that case, a species is defined as a separately evolving lineage that forms a single gene pool. Although properties such as DNA-sequences and morphology are used to help separate closely related lineages,[5] this definition has fuzzy boundaries.[6] However, the exact definition of the term "species" is still controversial, particularly in prokaryotes,[7] and this is called the species problem.[8] Biologists have proposed a range of more precise definitions, but the definition used is a pragmatic choice that depends on the particularities of the species of concern.[8]

Common names and species

The commonly used names for plant and animal taxa sometimes correspond to species: for example, "lion", "walrus", and "Camphor tree" – each refers to a species. In other cases common names do not: for example, "deer" refers to a family of 34 species, including Eld's Deer, Red Deer and Elk (Wapiti). The last two species were once considered a single species, illustrating how species boundaries may change with increased scientific knowledge.

Placement within genera

Ideally, a species is given a formal, scientific name, although in practice there are very many unnamed species (which have only been described, not named). When a species is named, it is placed within a genus. From a scientific point of view this can be regarded as a hypothesis that the species is more closely related to other species within its genus (if any) than to species of other genera. Species and genus are usually defined as part of a larger taxonomic hierarchy. The best-known taxonomic ranks are, in order: life, domain, kingdom, phylum, class, order, family, genus, and species. This assignment to a genus is not immutable; later a different (or the same) taxonomist may assign it to a different genus, in which case the name will also change.

In biological nomenclature, the name for a species is a two-part name (a binomial name), treated as Latin, although roots from any language can be used as well as names of locales or individuals. The generic name is listed first (with its leading letter capitalized), followed by a second term. The terminology used for the second term differs between zoological and botanical nomenclature.

- In zoological nomenclature, the second part of the name can be called the specific name or the specific epithet. For example, gray wolves belong to the species *Canis lupus*, coyotes to *Canis latrans*, golden jackals to *Canis aureus*, etc., and all of those belong to the genus *Canis* (which also contains many other species). For the gray wolf, the genus name is *Canis*, the specific name or specific epithet is *lupus*, and the binomen, the name of the species, is *Canis lupus*.
- In botanical nomenclature, the second part of the name can only be called the specific epithet. The 'specific name' in botany is always the combination of genus name and specific epithet. For example, the species commonly known as the longleaf pine is *Pinus palustris*; the genus name is *Pinus*, the specific epithet is *palustris*, the specific name is *Pinus palustris*.

This binomial naming convention, later formalized in the biological codes of nomenclature, was first used by Leonhart Fuchs and introduced as the standard by Carolus Linnaeus in his 1753, *Species Plantarum* (followed by his, 1758 *Systema Naturae*, 10th edition). At that time, the chief biological theory was that species represented independent acts of creation by God and were therefore considered objectively real and immutable, so the hypothesis of common descent did not apply.

Abbreviated names

Books and articles sometimes intentionally do not identify species fully and use the abbreviation "**sp.**" in the singular or "**spp.**" in the plural in place of the specific epithet: for example, ***Canis* sp.** This commonly occurs in the following types of situations:

- The authors are confident that some individuals belong to a particular genus but are not sure to which exact species they belong. This is particularly common in paleontology.
- The authors use "spp." as a short way of saying that something applies to many species within a genus, but do not wish to say that it applies to all species within that genus. If scientists mean that something applies to all species within a genus, they use the genus name without the specific epithet.

In books and articles, genus and species names are usually printed in italics. Abbreviations such as "sp.", "spp.", "subsp.", etc. should not be italicized.

Identification codes

Various codes have been devised for identifying particular species. For example:

- NCBI employs a numeric 'taxid' or *Taxonomy identifier*, a "stable unique identifier", e.g. the taxid of *H. sapiens* is 9606 [9]
- KEGG employs a three-letter code for a limited number of organisms; in this code, for example, *H. sapiens* is simply *hsa* [10];
- UniProt employs an "organism mnemonic" of not more than five alphanumeric characters, e.g. *HUMAN* for *H. sapiens* [11]

Difficulty of defining "species" and identifying particular species

It is surprisingly difficult to define the word "species" in a way that applies to all naturally occurring organisms, and the debate among biologists about how to define "species" and how to identify actual species is called the species problem. Over two dozen distinct definitions of "species" are in use amongst biologists.[12]

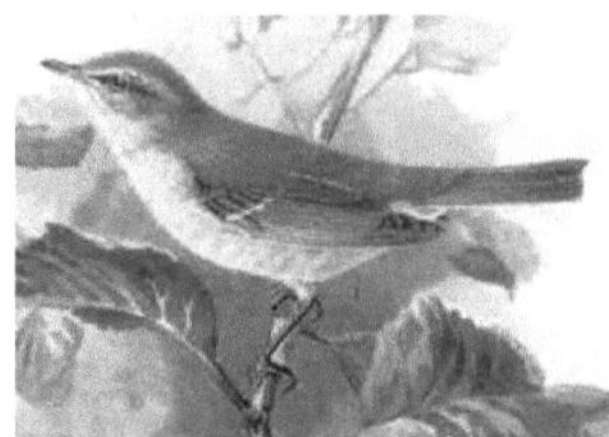

The Greenish Warbler demonstrates the concept of a ring species.

Most textbooks follow Ernst Mayr's definition of a species as "groups of actually or potentially interbreeding natural populations, which are reproductively isolated from other such groups".[8]

Various parts of this definition serve to exclude some unusual or artificial matings:

- Those that occur only in captivity (when the animal's normal mating partners may not be available) or as a result of deliberate human action
- Animals that may be physically and physiologically capable of mating but, for various reasons, do not normally do so in the wild

The typical textbook definition above works well for most multi-celled organisms, but there are several types of situations in which it breaks down:

- By definition it applies only to organisms that reproduce sexually. So it does not work for asexually reproducing single-celled organisms and for the relatively few parthenogenetic multi-celled organisms. The term "phylotype" is often applied to such organisms.
- Biologists frequently do not know whether two morphologically similar groups of organisms are "potentially" capable of interbreeding.
- There is considerable variation in the degree to which hybridization may succeed under natural conditions, or even in the degree to which some organisms use sexual reproduction between individuals to breed.
- In ring species, members of adjacent populations interbreed successfully but members of some non-adjacent populations do not.
- In a few cases it may be physically impossible for animals that are members of the same species to mate. However, these are cases, such as in breeds of dogs, in which human intervention has caused gross morphological changes, and are therefore excluded by the biological species concept.

Horizontal gene transfer makes it even more difficult to define the word "species". There is strong evidence of horizontal gene transfer between very dissimilar groups of prokaryotes, and at least occasionally between dissimilar groups of eukaryotes; and Williamson[13] argues that there is evidence for it in some crustaceans and echinoderms. All definitions of the word "species" assume that an organism gets all its genes from one or two parents that are very like that organism, but horizontal gene transfer makes that assumption false.

Definitions of species

The question of how best to define "species" is one that has occupied biologists for centuries, and the debate itself has become known as the species problem. Darwin wrote in chapter II of *On the Origin of Species*:

> No one definition has satisfied all naturalists; yet every naturalist knows vaguely what he means when he speaks of a species. Generally the term includes the unknown element of a distinct act of creation.[14]

But later, in *The Descent of Man*, when addressing "The question whether mankind consists of one or several species", Darwin revised his opinion to say:

> it is a hopeless endeavour to decide this point on sound grounds, until some definition of the term "species" is generally accepted; and the definition must not include an element that cannot possibly be ascertained, such as an act of creation.[15]

The modern theory of evolution depends on a fundamental redefinition of "species". Prior to Darwin, naturalists viewed species as ideal or general types, which could be exemplified by an ideal specimen bearing all the traits general to the species. Darwin's theories shifted attention from uniformity to variation and from the general to the particular. According to intellectual historian Louis Menand,

> Once our attention is redirected to the individual, we need another way of making generalizations. We are no longer interested in the conformity of an individual to an ideal type; we are now interested in the relation of an individual to the other individuals with which it interacts. To generalize about groups of interacting individuals, we need to drop the language of types and essences, which is prescriptive (telling us what finches should be), and adopt the language of statistics and probability, which is predictive (telling us what the average finch, under specified conditions, is likely to do). Relations will be more important than categories; functions, which are variable, will be more important than purposes; transitions will be more important than boundaries; sequences will be more important than hierarchies.[16]

This shift results in a new approach to "species"; Darwin concluded that species are what they appear to be: ideas, which are provisionally useful for naming groups of interacting individuals. "I look at the term species", he wrote, "as one arbitrarily given for the sake of convenience to a set of individuals closely resembling each other ... It does not essentially differ from the word variety, which is given to less distinct and more fluctuating forms. The term variety, again, in comparison with mere individual differences, is also applied arbitrarily, and for convenience sake." [16]

Practically, biologists define species as *populations of organisms that have a high level of genetic similarity*. This may reflect an adaptation to the same niche, and the transfer of genetic material from one individual to others, through a variety of possible means. The exact level of similarity used in such a definition is arbitrary, but this is the most common definition used for organisms that reproduce asexually (asexual reproduction), such as some plants and microorganisms.

This lack of any clear species concept in microbiology has led to some authors arguing that the term "species" is not useful when studying bacterial evolution. Instead they see genes as moving freely between even distantly related bacteria, with the entire bacterial domain being a single gene pool. Nevertheless, a kind of rule of thumb has been established, saying that species of *Bacteria* or *Archaea* with 16S rRNA gene sequences more similar than 97% to each other need to be checked by DNA-DNA Hybridization if they belong to the same species or not.[17] This concept has been updated recently, saying that the border of 97% was too low and can be raised to 98.7%.[18]

In the study of sexually reproducing organisms, where genetic material is shared through the process of reproduction, the ability of two organisms to interbreed and produce fertile offspring of both sexes is generally accepted as a simple indicator that the organisms share enough genes to be considered members of the same species. Thus a "species" is a group of interbreeding organisms.

This definition can be extended to say that a species is a group of organisms that could potentially interbreed – fish could still be classed as the same species even if they live in different lakes, as long as they could still interbreed were they ever to come into contact with each other. On the other hand, there are many examples of series of three or more distinct populations, where individuals of the population in the middle can interbreed with the populations to either side, but individuals of the populations on either side cannot interbreed. Thus, one could argue that these populations constitute a single species, or two distinct species. This is not a paradox; it is evidence that species are defined by gene frequencies, and thus have fuzzy boundaries.

Consequently, any single, universal definition of "species" is necessarily arbitrary. Instead, biologists have proposed a range of definitions; which definition a biologists uses is a pragmatic choice, depending on the particularities of that biologist's research.

In practice, these definitions often coincide, and the differences between them are more a matter of emphasis than of outright contradiction. Nevertheless, no species concept yet proposed is entirely objective, or can be applied in all cases without resorting to judgment. Given the complexity of life, some have argued that such an objective definition is in all likelihood impossible, and biologists should settle for the most practical definition.

For most vertebrates, this is the biological species concept (BSC), and to a lesser extent (or for different purposes) the phylogenetic species concept (PSC). Many BSC subspecies are considered species under the PSC; the difference between the BSC and the PSC can be summed up insofar as that the BSC defines a species as a consequence of manifest evolutionary *history*, while the PSC defines a species as a consequence of manifest evolutionary *potential*. Thus, a PSC species is "made" as soon as an evolutionary lineage has started to separate, while a BSC species starts to exist only when the lineage separation is complete. Accordingly, there can be considerable conflict between alternative classifications based upon the PSC versus BSC, as they differ completely in their treatment of taxa that would be considered subspecies under the latter model (e.g., the numerous subspecies of honey bees).

Typological species

A group of organisms in which individuals are members of the species if they sufficiently conform to certain fixed properties or "rights of passage". The clusters of variations or phenotypes within specimens (i.e. longer or shorter tails) would differentiate the species. This method was used as a "classical" method of determining species, such as with Linnaeus early in evolutionary theory. However, we now know that different phenotypes do not always constitute different species (e.g.: a 4-winged *Drosophila* born to a 2-winged mother is not a different species). Species named in this manner are called *morphospecies*.[19]

Evolutionary species

A single evolutionary lineage of organisms within which genes can be shared, and that maintains its integrity with respect to other lineages through both time and space. At some point in the evolution of such a group, some members may diverge from the main population and evolve into a subspecies, a process that may eventually lead to the formation of a new species if isolation (geographical or ecological) is maintained. A species that gives rise to another species is a paraphyletic species, or paraspecies. [20] [21]

Phylogenetic (cladistic) species

A group of organisms that shares an ancestor; a lineage that maintains its integrity with respect to other lineages through both time and space. At some point in the progress of such a group, members may diverge from one another: when such a divergence becomes sufficiently clear, the two populations are regarded as separate species. This differs from evolutionary species in that the parent species goes extinct taxonomically when a new species evolve, the mother and daughter populations now forming two new species.[22] Subspecies as such are not recognized under this approach; either a population is a phylogenetic species or it is not taxonomically distinguishable.

Other

Ecological species

A set of organisms adapted to a particular set of resources, called a niche, in the environment. According to this concept, populations form the discrete phenetic clusters that we recognize as species because the ecological and evolutionary processes controlling how resources are divided up tend to produce those clusters.[23]

Biological / reproductive species

Two organisms that are able to reproduce naturally to produce fertile offspring of both sexes. Organisms that can reproduce but almost always make infertile hybrids of at least one sex, such as a mule, hinny or F1 male cattalo are not considered to be the same species.

Biological / Isolation species

A set of actually or potentially interbreeding populations. This is generally a useful formulation for scientists working with living examples of the higher taxa like mammals, fish, and birds, but more problematic for organisms that do not reproduce sexually. The results of breeding experiments done in artificial conditions may or may not reflect what would happen if the same organisms encountered each other in the wild, making it difficult to gauge whether or not the results of such experiments are meaningful in reference to natural populations.

Genetic species

Based on similarity of DNA of individuals or populations. Techniques to compare similarity of DNA include DNA-DNA hybridization, and genetic fingerprinting (or DNA barcoding).

Cohesion species

Most inclusive population of individuals having the potential for phenotypic cohesion through intrinsic cohesion mechanisms. This is an expansion of the mate-recognition species concept to allow for post-mating isolation mechanisms; no matter whether populations can hybridize successfully, they are still distinct cohesion species if the amount of hybridization is insufficient to completely mix their respective gene pools.

Evolutionarily Significant Unit (ESU)

An evolutionarily significant unit is a population of organisms that is considered distinct for purposes of conservation. Often referred to as a species or a *wildlife species*, an ESU also has several possible definitions, which coincide with definitions of species.

Morphological species

A population or group of populations that differs morphologically from other populations. For example, we can distinguish between a chicken and a duck because they have different shaped bills and the duck has webbed feet. Species have been defined in this way since well before the beginning of recorded history. This species concept is highly criticized because more recent genetic data reveal that genetically distinct populations may look very similar and, contrarily, large morphological differences sometimes exist between very closely related populations. Nonetheless, most species known have been described solely from morphology.

Phenetic species

Based on phenotypes.

Microspecies

Species that reproduce without meiosis or fertilization so that each generation is genetically identical to the previous generation. See also apomixis.

Recognition species

Based on shared reproductive systems, including mating behavior. The Recognition concept of species has been introduced by Hugh E. H. Paterson, after earlier work by Wilhelm Petersen.

Mate-recognition species

A group of organisms that are known to recognize one another as potential mates. Like the isolation species concept above, it applies only to organisms that reproduce sexually. Unlike the isolation species concept, it focuses specifically on pre-mating reproductive isolation.

Numbers of species

Bearing in mind the aforementioned problems with categorising species, the following numbers are only a soft guide. In 2010, they broke down as follows:[24]

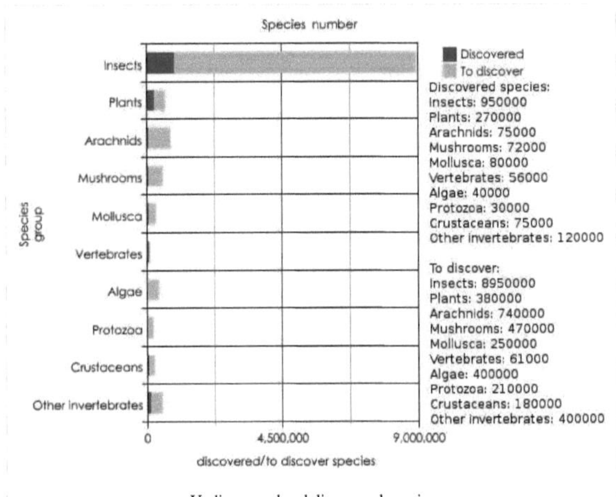

Undiscovered and discovered species

Total number of species (estimated): 7–100 million (identified and unidentified), including:

- 5–10 million bacteria;[25]
- 1.5 million fungi;[26]
- ~1 million mites[27]
- 10–30 million insects;[28]

Number of *identified* eukaryote species: 1.6 million, including:[29]

- 3,067 brown algae
- 321,212 plants, including:
  - 10,134 red and green algae
  - 16,236 mosses,
  - 12,000 ferns and horsetails,
  - 1,021 gymnosperms,
  - 281,821 angiosperms;
- 74,000-120,000 fungi;[26]
- 17,000 lichens;
- 1,367,555 animals, including:
  - 1,305,250 invertebrates
    - 2,175 corals
    - 85,000 mollusks
    - 102,248 arachnids
    - 47,000 crustaceans
    - 1,000,000 insects
    - 68,827 other invertebrates;
  - 62,305 vertebrates
    - 31,300 fish,
    - 6,433 amphibians,
    - 9,084 reptiles,
    - 9,998 birds,

- 5,490 mammals;

At present, organisations such as the Global Taxonomy Initiative, the European Distributed Institute of Taxonomy and the Census of Marine Life[30] (the latter only for marine organisms) are trying to improve taxonomy and implement previously undiscovered species to the taxonomy system. Because we know but a portion of the organisms in the biosphere, we do not have a complete understanding of the workings of our environment. To make matters worse, despite the discovery of new species, according to professor James Mallet, we are wiping out these species at an unprecedented rate.[31] This means that even before a new species has had the chance of being studied and classified, it may already be extinct.

Importance in biological classification

The idea of *species* has a long history. It is one of the most important levels of classification, for several reasons:

- It often corresponds to what lay people treat as the different basic kinds of organism – dogs are one species, cats another.
- It is the standard binomial nomenclature (or trinomial nomenclature) by which scientists typically refer to organisms.
- It is the highest taxonomic level that cannot be made more or less inclusionary.

After years of use, the concept remains central to biology and a host of related fields, and yet also remains at times ill-defined.

Implications of assignment of species status

The naming of a particular species may be regarded as a *hypothesis* about the evolutionary relationships and distinguishability of that group of organisms. As further information comes to hand, the hypothesis may be confirmed or refuted. Sometimes, especially in the past when communication was more difficult, taxonomists working in isolation have given two distinct names to individual organisms later identified as the same species. When two named species are discovered to be of the same species, the older species name is usually retained, and the newer species name dropped, a process called *synonymization*, or colloquially, as **lumping**. Dividing a taxon into multiple, often new, taxons is called **splitting**. Taxonomists are often referred to as "lumpers" or "splitters" by their colleagues, depending on their personal approach to recognizing differences or commonalities between organisms (see lumpers and splitters).

Traditionally, researchers relied on observations of anatomical differences, and on observations of whether different populations were able to interbreed successfully, to distinguish species; both anatomy and breeding behavior are still important to assigning species status. As a result of the revolutionary (and still ongoing) advance in microbiological research techniques, including DNA analysis, in the last few decades, a great deal of additional knowledge about the differences and similarities between species has become available. Many populations formerly regarded as separate species are now considered a single taxon, and many formerly grouped populations have been split. Any taxonomic level (species, genus, family, etc.) can be synonymized or split, and at higher taxonomic levels, these revisions have been still more profound.

From a taxonomical point of view, groups within a species can be defined as being of a taxon hierarchically lower than a species. In zoology only the subspecies is used, while in botany the variety, subvariety, and form are used as well. In conservation biology, the concept of evolutionary significant units (ESU) is used, which may define either species or smaller distinct population segments. Identifying and naming species is the providence of alpha taxonomy.

Historical development of the species concept

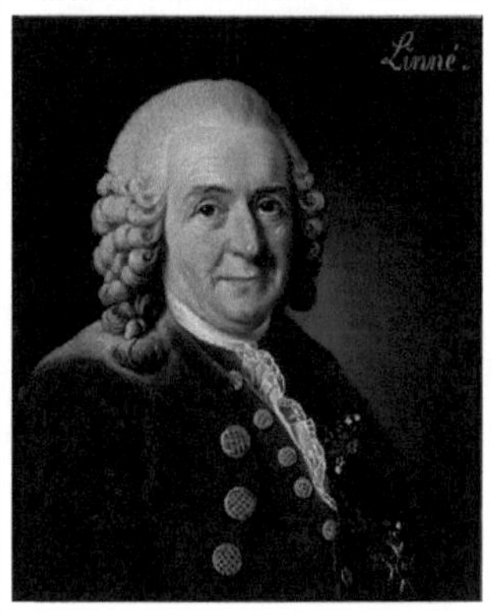

Linnaeus believed in the fixity of species.

In the earliest works of science, a species was simply an individual organism that represented a group of similar or nearly identical organisms. No other relationships beyond that group were implied. Aristotle used the words *genus* and *species* to mean generic and specific categories. Aristotle and other pre-Darwinian scientists took the species to be distinct and unchanging, with an "essence", like the chemical elements. When early observers began to develop systems of organization for living things, they began to place formerly isolated species into a context. Many of these early delineation schemes would now be considered whimsical and these included consanguinity based on color (all plants with yellow flowers) or behavior (snakes, scorpions and certain biting ants).

In the 18th century Swedish scientist Carolus Linnaeus classified organisms according to differences in the form of reproductive apparatus. Although his system of classification sorts organisms according to degrees of similarity, it made no claims about the relationship between similar species. At that time, it was still widely believed that there was no organic connection between species, no matter how similar they appeared. This approach also suggested a type of idealism: the notion that each species existed as an "ideal form". Although there are always differences (although sometimes minute) between individual organisms, Linnaeus considered such variation problematic. He strove to identify individual organisms that were exemplary of the species, and considered other non-exemplary organisms to be deviant and imperfect.

By the 19th century most naturalists understood that species could change form over time, and that the history of the planet provided enough time for major changes. Jean-Baptiste Lamarck, in his 1809 *Zoological Philosophy*, offered one of the first logical arguments against creationism. The new emphasis was on determining *how* a species could change over time. Lamarck suggested that an organism could pass on an acquired trait to its offspring, i.e., the giraffe's long neck was attributed to generations of giraffes stretching to reach the leaves of higher treetops (this well-known and simplistic example, however, does not do justice to the breadth and subtlety of Lamarck's ideas). With the acceptance of the natural selection idea of Charles Darwin in the 1860s, however, Lamarck's view of goal-oriented evolution, also known as a teleological process, was eclipsed. Recent interest in inheritance of acquired characteristics centers around epigenetic processes, e.g. methylation, that do not affect DNA sequences, but instead alter expression in an inheritable manner. Thus, neo-lamarckism, as it is sometimes termed, is not a challenge to the theory of evolution by natural selection.

Charles Darwin and Alfred Wallace provided what scientists now consider as the most powerful and compelling theory of evolution. Darwin argued that it was populations that evolved, not individuals. His argument relied on a radical shift in perspective from that of Linnaeus: rather than defining species in ideal terms (and searching for an ideal representative and rejecting deviations), Darwin considered variation among individuals to be natural. He further argued that variation, far from being problematic, actually provides the *explanation* for the existence of distinct species.

Darwin's work drew on Thomas Malthus' insight that the rate of growth of a biological population will always outpace the rate of growth of the resources in the environment, such as the food supply. As a result, Darwin argued, not all the members of a population will be able to survive and reproduce. Those that did will, on average, be the ones possessing variations—however slight—that make them slightly better adapted to the environment. If these variable traits are heritable, then the offspring of the survivors will also possess them. Thus, over many generations, adaptive variations will accumulate in the population, while counter-adaptive traits will tend to be eliminated.

Whether a variation is adaptive or non-adaptive depends on the environment: different environments favor different traits. Since the environment effectively selects which organisms live to reproduce, it is the environment (the "fight for existence") that selects the traits to be passed on. This is the theory of evolution by natural selection. In this model, the length of a giraffe's neck would be explained by positing that proto-giraffes with longer necks would have had a significant reproductive advantage to those with shorter necks. Over many generations, the entire population would be a species of long-necked animals.

In 1859, when Darwin published his theory of natural selection, the mechanism behind the inheritance of individual traits was unknown. Although Darwin made some speculations on how traits are inherited (pangenesis), his theory relies only on the fact that inheritable traits *exist*, and are variable (which makes his accomplishment even more remarkable.) Although Gregor Mendel's paper on genetics was published in 1866, its significance was not recognized. It was not until 1900 that his work was rediscovered by Hugo de Vries, Carl Correns and Erich von Tschermak, who realised that the "inheritable traits" in Darwin's theory are genes.

The theory of the evolution of species through natural selection has two important implications for discussions of species—consequences that fundamentally challenge the assumptions behind Linnaeus' taxonomy. First, it suggests that species are not just similar, they may actually be related. Some students of Darwin argue that *all* species are descended from a common ancestor. Second, it supposes that "species" are not homogeneous, fixed, permanent things; members of a species are all different, and over time species change. This suggests that species do not have any clear boundaries but are rather momentary statistical effects of constantly changing gene-frequencies. One may still use Linnaeus' taxonomy to identify individual plants and animals, but one can no longer think of species as independent and immutable.

The rise of a new species from a parental line is called speciation. There is no clear line demarcating the ancestral species from the descendant species.

Although the current scientific understanding of species suggests that there is no rigorous and comprehensive way to distinguish between different species in *all* cases, biologists continue to seek concrete ways to operationalize the idea. One of the most popular biological definitions of species is in terms of reproductive isolation; if two creatures cannot reproduce to produce fertile offspring of both sexes, then they are in different species. This definition captures a number of intuitive species boundaries, but it remains imperfect. It has nothing to say about species that reproduce asexually, for example, and it is very difficult to apply to extinct species. Moreover, boundaries between species are often fuzzy: there are examples where members of one population can produce fertile offspring of both sexes with a second population, and members of the second population can produce fertile offspring of both sexes with members of a third population, but members of the first and third population cannot produce fertile offspring, or can only produce fertile offspring of the homozygous sex. Consequently, some people reject this definition of a species.

Richard Dawkins defines two organisms as conspecific if and only if they have the same number of chromosomes and, for each chromosome, both organisms have the same number of nucleotides (*The Blind Watchmaker*, p. 118). However, most if not all taxonomists would strongly disagree. For example, in many amphibians, most notably in New Zealand's *Leiopelma* frogs, the genome consists of "core" chromosomes that are mostly invariable and accessory chromosomes, of which exist a number of possible combinations. Even though the chromosome numbers are highly variable between populations, these can interbreed successfully and form a single evolutionary unit. In plants, polyploidy is extremely commonplace with few restrictions on interbreeding; as individuals with an odd number of chromosome sets are usually sterile, depending on the actual number of chromosome sets present, this results in the odd situation where some individuals of the same evolutionary unit can interbreed with certain others and some cannot, with all populations being eventually linked as to form a common gene pool.

The classification of species has been profoundly affected by technological advances that have allowed researchers to determine relatedness based on molecular markers, starting with the comparatively crude blood plasma precipitation assays in the mid-20th century to Charles Sibley's ground-breaking DNA-DNA hybridization studies in the 1970s leading to DNA sequencing techniques. The results of these techniques caused revolutionary changes in the higher taxonomic categories (such as phyla and classes), resulting in the reordering of many branches of the phylogenetic tree (*see also:* molecular phylogeny). For taxonomic categories below genera, the results have been mixed so far; the pace of evolutionary change on the molecular level is rather slow, yielding clear differences only after considerable periods of reproductive separation. DNA-DNA hybridization results have led to misleading conclusions, the Pomarine Skua – Great Skua phenomenon being a famous example. Turtles have been determined to evolve with just one-eighth of the speed of other reptiles on the molecular level, and the rate of molecular evolution in albatrosses is half of what is found in the rather closely related storm-petrels. The hybridization technique is now obsolete and is replaced by more reliable computational approaches for sequence comparison. Molecular taxonomy is not directly based on the evolutionary processes, but rather on the overall change brought upon by these processes. The processes that lead to the generation and maintenance of variation such as mutation, crossover and selection are not uniform (see also molecular clock). DNA is only extremely rarely a direct target of natural selection rather than changes in the DNA sequence enduring over generations being a result of the latter; for example, silent transition-transversion combinations would alter the melting point of the DNA sequence, but not the sequence of the encoded proteins and thus are a possible example where, for example in microorganisms, a mutation confers a change in fitness all by itself.

See also

- Cline
- Cryptic species complex
- Encyclopedia of Life
- Endangered species
- Ring species
- Species naming
- Species problem
- Systematics

Notes and references

[1] Sahney, S., Benton, M.J. and Ferry, P.A. (2010). "Links between global taxonomic diversity, ecological diversity and the expansion of vertebrates on land" (http://rsbl.royalsocietypublishing.org/content/6/4/544.full.pdf+html) (PDF). *Biology Letters* **6** (4): 544–547. doi:10.1098/rsbl.2009.1024. PMC 2936204. PMID 20106856. .

[2] Sahney, S. and Benton, M.J. (2008). "Recovery from the most profound mass extinction of all time" (http://journals.royalsociety.org/content/qq5un1810k7605h5/fulltext.pdf) (PDF). *Proceedings of the Royal Society: Biological* **275** (1636): 759. doi:10.1098/rspb.2007.1370. PMC 2596898. PMID 18198148. .

[3] Goldenberg, Suzanne (2011-08-23). "Planet Earth is home to 8.7 million species, scientists estimate" (http://www.guardian.co.uk/environment/2011/aug/23/species-earth-estimate-scientists). *The Guardian* (London). . Retrieved 2011-08-23

[4] "Just How Many Species Are There, Anyway?" (http://www.sciencedaily.com/releases/2003/05/030526103731.htm). 2003-05-26. . Retrieved 2008-01-15

[5] Koch, H. 2010. Combining morphology and DNA barcoding resolves the taxonomy of Western Malagasy *Liotrigona* Moure, 1961. *African Invertebrates* **51** (2): 413-421. (http://www.africaninvertebrates.org.za/Koch_2010_51_2_474.aspx) PDF fulltext (http://www.tb1.ethz.ch/PublicationsEO/PDFpapers/Koch_AFRICAN_INVERTEBRATES_2010_51_413-421.pdf)

[6] De Queiroz K (December 2007). "Species concepts and species delimitation". *Syst. Biol.* **56** (6): 879–86. doi:10.1080/10635150701701083. PMID 18027281.

[7] Fraser C, Alm EJ, Polz MF, Spratt BG, Hanage WP (February 2009). "The bacterial species challenge: making sense of genetic and ecological diversity". *Science* **323** (5915): 741–6. doi:10.1126/science.1159388. PMID 19197054.

[8] de Queiroz K (May 2005). "Ernst Mayr and the modern concept of species" (http://www.pnas.org/cgi/pmidlookup?view=long&pmid=15851674). *Proc. Natl. Acad. Sci. U.S.A.* **102** (Suppl 1): 6600–7. doi:10.1073/pnas.0502030102. PMC 1131873. PMID 15851674. .

[9] http://www.ncbi.nlm.nih.gov/Taxonomy

[10] http://www.genome.jp/kegg/catalog/org_list.html

[11] http://www.uniprot.org/help/taxonomy

[12] Wilkins, John (2010-10-20). "How many species concepts are there?" (http://www.guardian.co.uk/science/punctuated-equilibrium/2010/oct/20/3). London: *The Guardian*. . Retrieved 2010-10-19.

[13] David I. Williamson (2003). *The Origins of Larvae*. Kluwer. ISBN 1-4020-1514-3.

[14] Darwin 1859 p.59 (http://darwin-online.org.uk/content/frameset?viewtype=side&itemID=F373&pageseq=59)

[15] Darwin 1871 p. 24 (http://darwin-online.org.uk/content/frameset?viewtype=text&itemID=F937.1&keywords=definition+species+of&pageseq=241)

[16] Menand, Louis (2001). *The Metaphysical Club: A Story of Ideas in America*. Farrar, Straus and Giroux. pp. 123–124.

[17] Stackebrandt E, Goebel BM (1994). "Taxonomic note: a place for DNA-DNA reassociation and 16S rRNA sequence analysis in the present species definition in bacteriology". *Int. J. Syst. Bacteriol.* **44**: 846–9. doi:10.1099/00207713-44-4-846.

[18] Stackebrandt E, Ebers J (2006). "Taxonomic parameters revisited: tarnished gold standards". *Microbiol. Today* **33**: 152–5.

[19] Michael Ruse (August 1969). "Definitions of Species in Biology". *The British Journal for the Philosophy of Science* (Oxford University Press) **20** (2): 97–119. doi:10.1093/bjps/20.2.97. JSTOR 686173.

[20] Paraspecies

[21] James S. Albert; Roberto E. Reis. *Historical Biogeography of Neotropical Freshwater Fishes* (http://books.google.com/books?id=V8kZeHxkv9oC&pg=PA316&lpg=PA316&dq=evolutionary+species+concept+Alberty+Reis&source=bl&ots=Qd1DbXoGJv&sig=FausTKz_R9mhDEzHMpbk9Tq61K0&hl=en&ei=BipcTu-gIsq2twfM9PigDA&sa=X&oi=book_result&ct=result&resnum=1&ved=0CCAQ6AEwAA#v=onepage&q&f=false). .

[22] Ereshefsky M (2002). "Linnean ranks: vestiges of a bygone era". *Philosophy of Science* **69**: S305–S315. JSTOR 10.

[23] Ridley, Mark. "The Idea of Species". *Evolution* (2nd ed.). Blackwell Science. p. 410. ISBN 0-86542-495-0.

[24] Current Results– Number of Species on Earth (http://www.currentresults.com/Environment-Facts/Plants-Animals/number-species.php)

[25] Sogin ML, Morrison HG, Huber JA, *et al.* (August 2006). "Microbial diversity in the deep sea and the underexplored "rare biosphere"" (http://www.pnas.org/cgi/pmidlookup?view=long&pmid=16880384). *Proc. Natl. Acad. Sci. U.S.A.* **103** (32): 12115–20. doi:10.1073/pnas.0605127103. PMC 1524930. PMID 16880384. . Cheung L (Monday, 31 July 200). "Thousands of microbes in one gulp" (http://news.bbc.co.uk/1/hi/sci/tech/5232928.stm). BBC. .

[26] David L. Hawksworth (2001). "The magnitude of fungal diversity: the 1•5 million species estimate revisited" (http://journals.cambridge.org/action/displayAbstract?fromPage=online&aid=95069). *Mycological Research* **105** (12): 1422–1432. doi:10.1017/S0953756201004725.
.

[27] Acari at University of Michigan Museum of Zoology Web Page (http://insects.ummz.lsa.umich.edu/ACARI/index.html)

[28] Encyclopedia Smithsonian: Numbers of Insects (http://www.si.edu/Encyclopedia_SI/nmnh/buginfo/bugnos.htm)

[29] "Number of Species on Earth" (http://www.currentresults.com/Environment-Facts/Plants-Animals/number-species.php). Current Results. 2007-01-01. . Retrieved 2010-04-23.

[30] "Census of marine life" (http://www.coml.org/). Coml.org. . Retrieved 2010-04-23.

[31] Robin McKie and Zoe Corbyn (2005-09-25). "Discovery of new species and extermination at high rate" (http://www.guardian.co.uk/science/2005/sep/25/taxonomy.conservationandendangeredspecies). London: Guardian. . Retrieved 2010-04-23.

External links

- Stanford Encyclopedia of Philosophy entry: *Species* (http://plato.stanford.edu/entries/species/)
- Barcoding of species (http://www.barcodinglife.org/)
- European Species Names in Linnaean, Czech, English, German and French (http://www.finitesite.com/dandelion/Linnaeus.HTML)
- Catalogue of Life (http://www.catalogueoflife.org/)
- VisualTaxa (http://visualtaxa.redgolpe.com/)
- Speciation (http://users.rcn.com/jkimball.ma.ultranet/BiologyPages/S/Speciation.html)

Articles online

- Other Species Concepts (http://evolution.berkeley.edu/evosite/evo101/VA2OtherSpeciesConcept.shtml) - *U.C. Berkeley*
- "Gone" (http://www.motherjones.com/news/feature/2007/05/gone.html), *Mother Jones*, May/June 2007.
- 2003-12-31, ScienceDaily: Working On The 'Porsche Of Its Time': New Model For Species Determination Offered (http://www.sciencedaily.com/releases/2003/12/031231082553.htm)
- 2003-08-08, ScienceDaily: Cross-species Mating May Be Evolutionarily Important And Lead To Rapid Change (http://www.sciencedaily.com/releases/2003/08/030808081854.htm)
- 2004-01-09 ScienceDaily: Mayo Researchers Observe Genetic Fusion Of Human, Animal Cells; May Help Explain Origin Of AIDS (http://www.sciencedaily.com/releases/2004/01/040109064407.htm)

- 2000-09-18, ScienceDaily: Scientists Unravel Ancient Evolutionary History Of Photosynthesis (http://www.sciencedaily.com/releases/2000/09/000913211733.htm)

Domain_(biology)

In biological taxonomy, a **domain** (also **superregnum**, **superkingdom**, **empire**, or **regio**) is the highest taxonomic rank of organisms, higher than a kingdom. According to the three-domain system of Carl Woese, introduced in 1990, the Tree of Life consists of three domains: Archaea, Bacteria and Eukarya.[1] The arrangement of taxa reflects the fundamental differences in the genomes. Alternative classifications of life so far proposed include:

- The two-empire system or **superdomain system**, with top-level groupings of Prokaryota (or Monera) and Eukaryota.[2] [3]
- The six-kingdom system with top-level groupings of Eubacteria, Archaebacteria, Protista, Fungi, Plantae, and Animalia.
- The three-empire system (Eubacteria, Archaea, Eukarya) with five **supergroups** in the Eukarya (Unikonta, Excavata, Chromalveolata, Rhizaria and Archaeplastida)[2] [4] [5]

None of the three systems currently include non-cellular life.

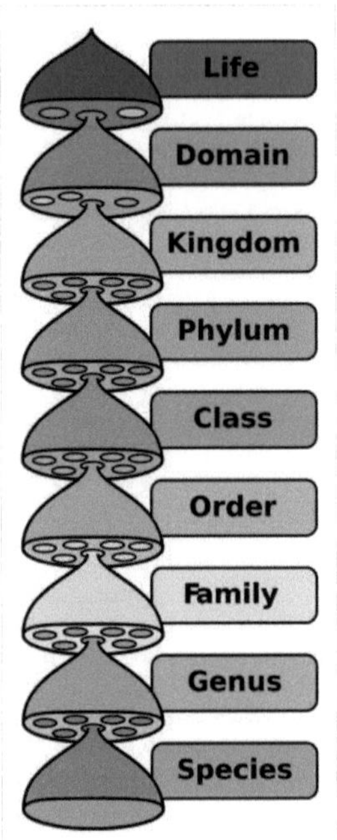

The hierarchy of biological classification's eight major taxonomic ranks, which is an example of definition by genus and differentia. Life is divided into domains, which are subdivided into further groups. Intermediate minor rankings are not shown.

See also

- Phylogenetics
- Systematics

References

[1] Woese C, Kandler O, Wheelis M (1990). "Towards a natural system of organisms: proposal for the domains Archaea, Bacteria, and Eucarya." (http://www.pnas.org/cgi/reprint/87/12/4576). *Proc Natl Acad Sci USA* **87** (12): 4576–9. Bibcode 1990PNAS...87.4576W. doi:10.1073/pnas.87.12.4576. PMC 54159. PMID 2112744. . Retrieved 11 February 2010.

[2] Mayr, Ernst (1998). "Two empires or three?." (http://www.pnas.org/content/95/17/9720.full). *Proc Natl Acad Sci USA* **95** (17): 9720–9723. Bibcode 1998PNAS...95.9720. doi:10.1073/pnas.95.17.9720. . Retrieved 5 Sept 2011.

[3] Cavalier-Smith, T. (2004), "Only six kingdoms of life" (http://www.cladocera.de/protozoa/cavalier-smith_2004_prs.pdf), *Proc. R. Soc. Lond. B* **271**: 1251–62, doi:10.1098/rspb.2004.2705, PMC 1691724, PMID 15306349, , retrieved 2010-04-29

[4] Campbell, N. A., et al. (2008) "Biology." 8th edition. *Person International Edition, San Francisco*

[5] Holt, Jack R. and Carlos A. Iudica, (2010) "Taxa of Life." (http://comenius.susqu.edu/bi/202/Taxa.htm) Retrieved 09-03-2011.

Juglandaceae

Juglandaceae	
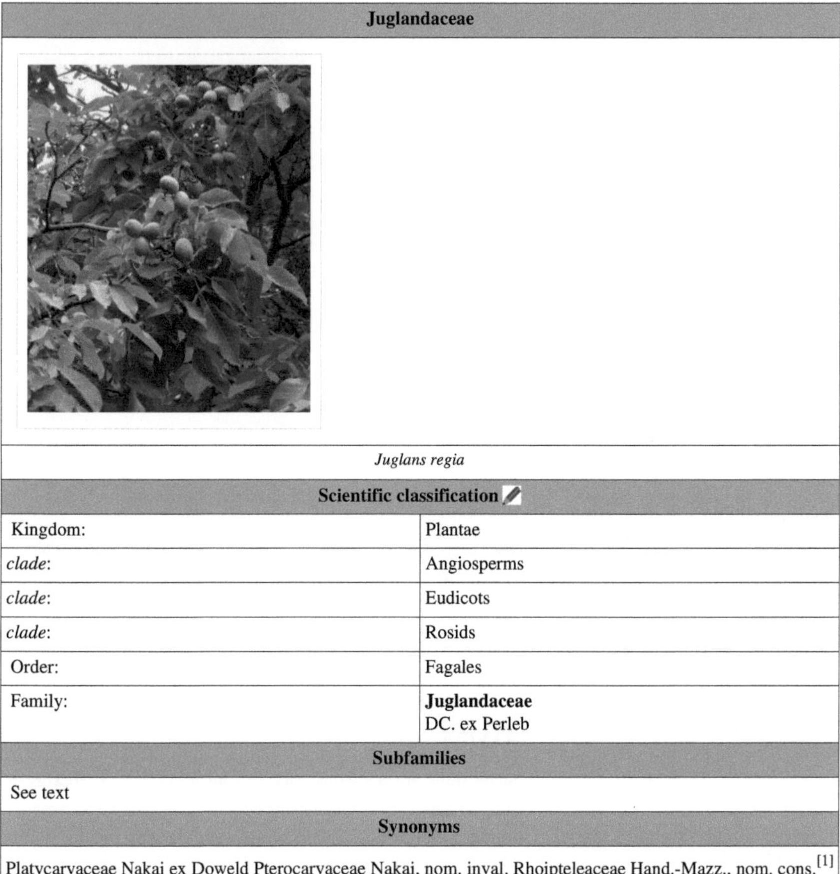	
Juglans regia	
Scientific classification	
Kingdom:	Plantae
clade:	Angiosperms
clade:	Eudicots
clade:	Rosids
Order:	Fagales
Family:	**Juglandaceae** DC. ex Perleb
Subfamilies	
See text	
Synonyms	
Platycaryaceae Nakai ex Doweld Pterocaryaceae Nakai, nom. inval. Rhoipteleaceae Hand.-Mazz., nom. cons.[1]	

The **Juglandaceae**, also known as the walnut family, is a family of trees, or sometimes shrubs, in the order Fagales. Various members of this family are native to the Americas, Eurasia, and Southeast Asia. Members of the walnut family have large, aromatic leaves that are usually alternate, but opposite in *Alfaroa* and *Oreomunnia*. The leaves are pinnately compound, or ternate, and usually 20–100 cm long.

The trees are wind-pollinated, and the flowers are usually arranged in catkins.

The eight genera in the family include the commercially important nut-producing trees walnut (*Juglans*), pecan (*Carya illinoinensis*), and hickory (*Carya*). The Persian walnut, *Juglans regia*, is one of the major nut crops of the world. Walnut, hickory, and gaulin are also valuable timber trees.

Systematics

The known living genera are grouped into subfamilies, tribes, and subtribes as follows:[2]

Subfamily Engelhardioideae

- *Alfaroa* Standl. – gaulin
- *Engelhardia* Lesch. ex Blume – cheo
- *Oreomunnea* Oerst.

Subfamily Juglandoideae

Tribe Platycaryeae

- *Platycarya* Siebold & Zucc.

Tribe Juglandeae

Subtribe Caryinae

- *Carya* Nutt. – hickory and pecan
- *Annamocarya* A.Chev.

Subtribe Juglandinae

- *Cyclocarya* Iljinsk – wheel wingnut
- *Juglans* L. – walnut
- *Pterocarya* Kunth – wingnut

Incertae sedis

- *Rhoiptelea* Diels & Hand.-Mazz.[3]

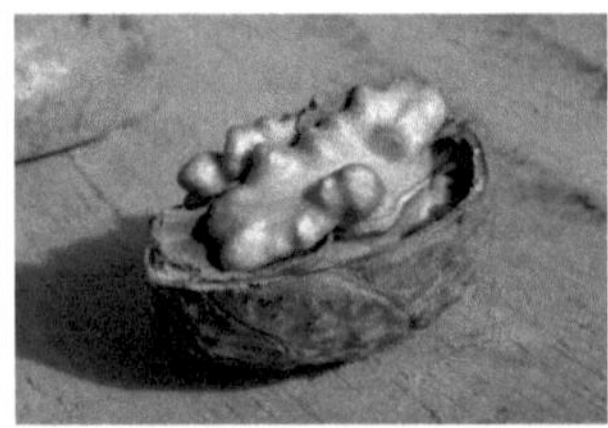

Nut of *Juglans regia*

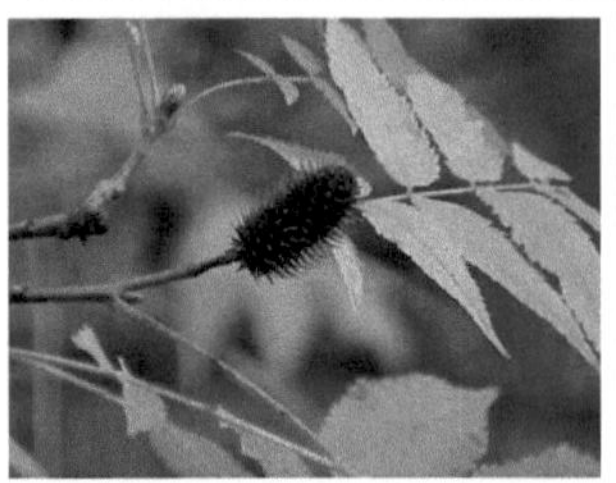

Foliage and seed catkin of *Platycarya strobilacea*

The only member of the genus *Alfaropsis* I.A.Iljinsk., *Alfaropsis roxburghiana* (Wall.) I.A.Iljinsk. is a synonym for *Engelhardia roxburghiana* Wall. (or perhaps vice-versa).

The only member of the genus *Annamocarya* A.Chev., *Annamocarya sinensis* (Dode) J.-F.Leroy, may actually be a member of *Carya*.

Tryma

Some fruits are borderline and difficult to categorize. Hickory nuts (*Carya*) and walnuts (*Juglans*) grow within an outer husk; these fruits are technically drupes or drupaceous nuts, and thus not true botanical nuts. "Tryma" is a specialized term for such nut-like drupes.[4] [5]

References

[1] "Family: *Juglandaceae* DC. ex Perleb, nom. cons." (http://www.ars-grin.gov/cgi-bin/npgs/html/family.pl?595). *Germplasm Resources Information Network*. United States Department of Agriculture. 2003-01-17. . Retrieved 2011-11-17.

[2] Manos, P. S.; D. E. Stone (2001). "Evolution, phylogeny and systematics of the Juglandaceae". *Annals of the Missouri Botanical Garden* **88**: 231–269.

[3] "GRIN Genera of *Juglandaceae*" (http://www.ars-grin.gov/cgi-bin/npgs/html/gnlist.pl?595). *Germplasm Resources Information Network*. United States Department of Agriculture. . Retrieved 2011-11-17.

[4] Armstrong, W.P.. "Identification Of Major Fruit Types" (http://waynesword.palomar.edu/fruitid1.htm). Wayne's World. . Retrieved 2011-11-17.

[5] Armstrong, W.P. (2009-03-15). "Fruits Called Nuts" (http://waynesword.palomar.edu/ecoph8.htm). Wayne's World. . Retrieved 2011-11-17.

Hickory

Hickory	
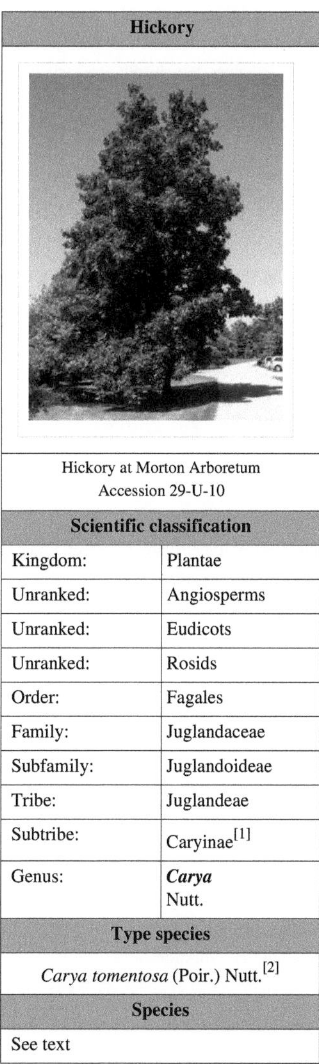	
Hickory at Morton Arboretum Accession 29-U-10	
Scientific classification	
Kingdom:	Plantae
Unranked:	Angiosperms
Unranked:	Eudicots
Unranked:	Rosids
Order:	Fagales
Family:	Juglandaceae
Subfamily:	Juglandoideae
Tribe:	Juglandeae
Subtribe:	Caryinae[1]
Genus:	***Carya*** Nutt.
Type species	
Carya tomentosa (Poir.) Nutt.[2]	
Species	
See text	

Trees in the genus ***Carya*** (Greek: κάρυον "nut") are commonly known as **hickory**, derived from the Powhatan language of Virginia. The genus includes 17–19 species of deciduous trees with pinnately compound leaves and big nuts. Five or six species are native to China, Indochina, and India (State of Assam), 11 or 12 are from the United States, two to four are from Canada and four are found in Mexico.

Another Asian species, **beaked hickory**, previously listed as *Carya sinensis*, is now treated in a separate genus, *Annamocarya*, as *Annamocarya sinensis*.

Hickory flowers are small, yellow-green catkins produced in spring. They are wind-pollinated and self-incompatible. The fruit is a globose or oval nut, 2–5 cm (**unknown operator: u'strong'unknown operator: u'strong'unknown operator: u'strong' unknown operator: u'strong'**) long and 1.5–3 cm (**unknown operator: u'strong'unknown operator: u'strong'unknown operator: u'strong' unknown operator: u'strong'**) diameter, enclosed in a four-valved husk, which splits open at maturity. The nut shell is thick and bony in most species, and thin in a few, notably *C. illinoinensis*; it is divided into two halves, which split apart when the seed germinates.

Species and classification

In the APG system, genus *Carya* (and the whole Juglandaceae family) has been recently moved to the Fagales order.

Asia

- ***Carya* sect. *Sinocarya*** – Asian hickories
  - *Carya dabieshanensis* M.C. Liu – Dabie Shan Hickory (may be synonymous with *C. cathayensis*)
  - *Carya cathayensis* Sarg. – Chinese Hickory
  - *Carya hunanensis* W.C.Cheng & R.H.Chang – Hunan Hickory
  - *Carya kweichowensis* Kuang & A.M.Lu – Guizhou Hickory
  - *Carya poilanei* Leroy - Poilane's Hickory
  - *Carya tonkinensis* Lecomte – Vietnamese Hickory[3]

North America

- ***Carya* sect. *Carya*** – typical hickories
  - *Carya floridana* Sarg. – Scrub Hickory
  - *Carya glabra* (Mill.) Sweet – Pignut Hickory, Pignut, Sweet Pignut, Coast Pignut Hickory, Smoothbark Hickory, Swamp Hickory, Broom Hickory
  - *Carya myristiciformis* (F.Michx.) Nutt. – Nutmeg Hickory, Swamp Hickory, Bitter Water Hickory
  - *Carya ovalis* (Wangenh.) Sarg. – Red Hickory, Spicebark Hickory, Sweet Pignut Hickory (treated as a synonym of *C. glabra* by *Flora N. Amer.*)
  - *Carya ovata* (Mill.) K.Koch – Shagbark Hickory
    - *Carya ovata var. ovata* – Northern Shagbark Hickory
    - *Carya ovata var. australis* – Southern Shagbark Hickory, Carolina Hickory (syn. *C. carolinae-septentrionalis*)
  - *Carya laciniosa* (Mill.) K.Koch – Shellbark Hickory, Shagbark Hickory, Bigleaf Shagbark Hickory, Kingnut, Big Shellbark, Bottom Shellbark, Thick Shellbark, Western Shellbark
  - *Carya pallida* (Ashe) Engl. & Graebn. – Sand Hickory
  - *Carya texana* Buckley – Black Hickory
  - *Carya tomentosa* (Poir.) Nutt. – Mockernut Hickory (syn. *C. alba*)
  - †*Carya washingtonensis* - Manchester Extinct Miocene
- ***Carya* sect. *Apocarya*** – pecans
  - *Carya aquatica* (F.Michx.) Nutt. – Bitter pecan or Water Hickory
  - *Carya cordiformis* (Wangenh.) K.Koch – Bitternut Hickory
  - *Carya illinoinensis* (Wangenh.) K.Koch – Pecan
  - *Carya palmeri* W.E. Manning – Mexican Hickory

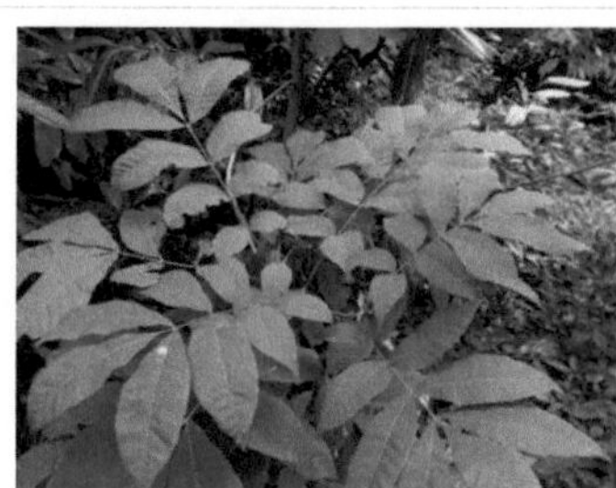

Carya cordiformis (bitternut hickory) foliage

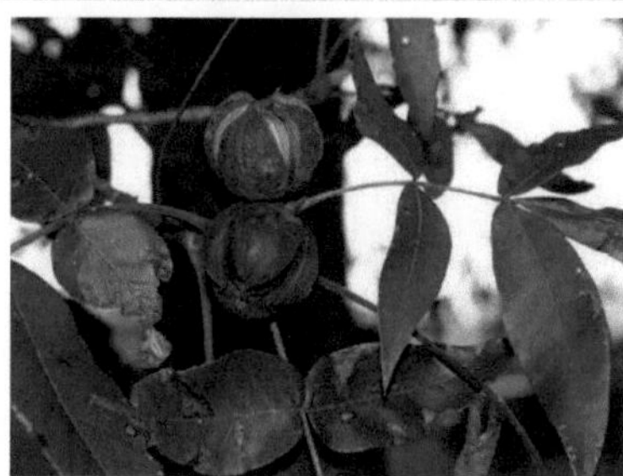

Ripe hickory nuts ready to fall, Andrews, SC

Ecology

Hickory is used as a food plant by the larvae of some Lepidoptera species. These include:

- Luna moth (*Actias luna*)
- Brown-tail (*Euproctis chrysorrhoea*)
- *Coleophora* case-bearers, *C. laticornella* and *C. ostryae*
- Regal moths (*Citheronia regalis*), whose caterpillars are known as hickory horn-devils
- Walnut sphinx (*Amorpha juglandis*)
- The Bride (nominate subspecies *Catocala neogama neogama*)

The hickory leaf stem gall phylloxera (*Phylloxera caryaecaulis*) also uses the hickory tree as a food source. Phylloxeridae are related to aphids and have a similarly complex life cycle. Eggs hatch in early spring and the galls quickly form around the developing insects. *Phylloxera* galls may damage weakened or stressed hickories, but are generally harmless. Deformed leaves and twigs can rain down from the tree in the spring as squirrels break off infected tissue and eat the galls, possibly for the protein content or because the galls are fleshy and tasty to the squirrels.

The banded hickory borer (*Knulliana cincta*) is also found on hickories.

Tryma

Some fruits are borderline and difficult to categorize. Hickory nuts (*Carya*) and walnuts (*Juglans*) in the Juglandaceae family grow within an outer husk; these fruits are technically drupes or drupaceous nuts, and thus not true botanical nuts. "Tryma" is a specialized term for such nut-like drupes.[4] [5]

Uses

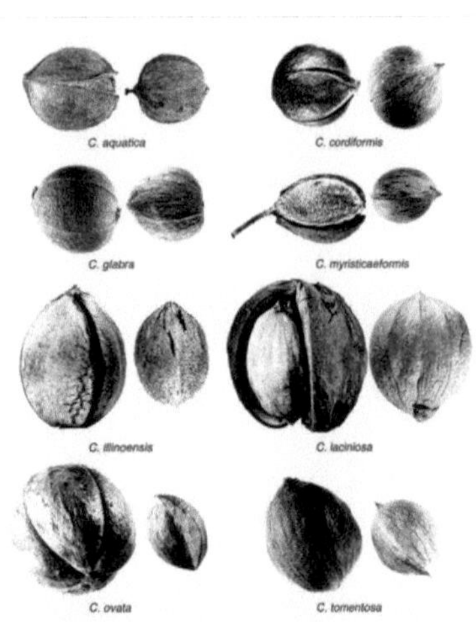

Comparison of North American *Carya* nuts

Hickory wood is very hard, stiff, dense and shock resistant. There are woods that are stronger than hickory and woods that are harder, but the combination of strength, toughness, hardness, and stiffness found in hickory wood is not found in any other commercial wood.[6] It is used for tool handles, bows, wheel spokes, carts, drumsticks, lacrosse stick handles, golf club shafts (sometimes still called *hickory stick*, even though made of steel or graphite), the bottom of skis, walking sticks and for punitive use as a switch (like hazel), and especially as a cane-like hickory stick in schools and use by parents. Paddles are often made from hickory. Baseball bats were formerly made of hickory, but are now more commonly made of ash. Hickory is replacing ash as the wood of choice for Scottish shinty sticks (also known as camans). Hickory was extensively used for the construction of early aircraft.

Hickory is also highly prized for wood-burning stoves, because of its high energy content. Hickory wood is also a preferred type for smoking cured meats. In the Southern United States, hickory is popular for cooking barbecue, as hickory grows abundantly in the region, and adds flavor to the meat. Hickory is sometimes used for wood flooring due to its durability and character.

A bark extract from shagbark hickory is also used in an edible syrup similar to maple syrup, with a slightly bitter, smoky taste.

The nuts of some species are palatable, while others are bitter and only suitable for animal feed. Shagbark and shellbark hickory, along with pecan, are regarded by some as the finest nut trees.

When cultivated for their nuts, clonal (grafted) trees of the same cultivar cannot pollinate each other because of their self-incompatibility. Two or more cultivars must be planted together for successful pollination. Seedlings (grown from hickory nuts) will usually have sufficient genetic variation.

See also

- Walnut
- Hican

References

[1] "Evolution, phylogeny and systematics of the Juglandaceae". *Annals of the Missouri Botanical Garden* **88**: 231–269. 2001.

[2] "*Carya* Nutt." (http://www.tropicos.org/Name/40002070). *TROPICOS*. Missouri Botanical Garden. . Retrieved 2009-10-19.

[3] "Subordinate Taxa of *Carya* Nutt." (http://www.tropicos.org/NameSubordinateTaxa.aspx?nameid=40002070). *TROPICOS*. Missouri Botanical Garden. . Retrieved 2009-10-19.

[4] Identification Of Major Fruit Types (http://waynesword.palomar.edu/fruitid1.htm)

[5] Fruits Called Nuts (http://waynesword.palomar.edu/ecoph8.htm)

[6] Important Trees of Eastern Forests, USDA, 1974

Bibliography

Philips, Roger. Trees of North America and Europe, Random House, Inc., New York ISBN 0-394-50259-0, 1979.

External links

- Flora of North America: *Carya* (http://www.efloras.org/florataxon.aspx?flora_id=1&taxon_id=105766)
- Flora of China: *Carya* (http://www.efloras.org/florataxon.aspx?flora_id=2&taxon_id=105766)
- USDA Agricultural Research Service: *Carya* (http://extension-horticulture.tamu.edu/carya/species/index.htm)
- Edibility of different species' nuts, from a snack food manufacturer (http://www.thenutfactory.com/kitchen/edible/facts-hickories.html)
- Comparison of eastern North American hickories at bioimages.vanderbilt.edu (http://www.cas.vanderbilt.edu/bioimages/pages/compare-hickories.htm)
- Comparison of hickory nuts at bioimages.vanderbilt.edu (http://www.cas.vanderbilt.edu/bioimages/pages/carya-fruits.htm)
- USDA Plants Database Profile for Carya (hickory) (http://plants.usda.gov/java/profile?symbol=CARYA)
- The northern shagbark hickory (http://www.songonline.ca/ecsong/northern_shags/index.html)

Taxonomic_rank

In biological classification, **rank** is the level (the relative position) in a taxonomic hierarchy. Examples of taxonomic ranks are species, genus, family, and class.

Each rank subsumes under it a number of less general categories. The rank of *species*, and specification of the *genus* to which the species belongs is *basic*, which means that it may not be necessary to specify ranks other than these.[1]

The *International Code of Zoological Nomenclature* defines rank as:

> The level, for nomenclatural purposes, of a taxon in a taxonomic hierarchy (e.g. all families are for nomenclatural purposes at the same rank, which lies between superfamily and subfamily)[2]

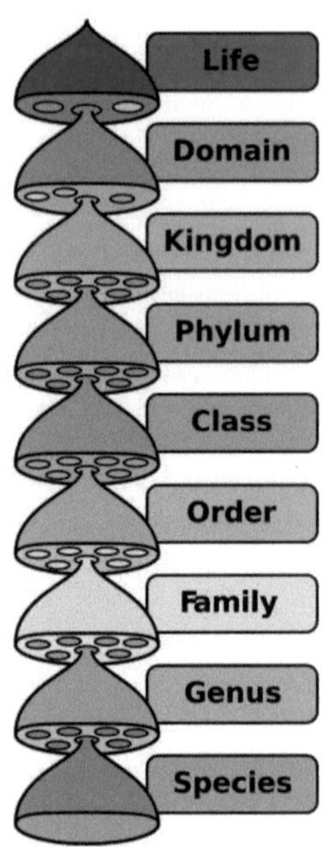

The hierarchy of biological classification's eight major taxonomic ranks, which is an example of definition by genus and differentia. Intermediate minor rankings are not shown.

Main ranks

"2.1. Every individual plant is treated as belonging to an indefinite number of taxa of consecutively subordinate rank, among which the rank of species (species) is basic."

In his landmark publications, such as the *Systema Naturae*, Carolus Linnaeus used a ranking scale limited to: kingdom, class, order, genus, species, and one rank below species. Today, nomenclature is regulated by the nomenclature codes, which allow names divided into an indefinite number of ranks. There are seven main taxonomic ranks: kingdom, phylum or division, class, order, family, genus, species. In addition, the *domain* (proposed by Carl Woese) is now widely used as one of the fundamental ranks, although it is not mentioned in any of the nomenclature codes.

Main taxonomic ranks			
Latin		English	
regio		domain	
regnum		kingdom	
phylum	*divisio*	phylum (in zoology)	division (in botany)
classis		class	
ordo		order	
familia		family	
genus		genus	
species		species	

A taxon is usually assigned a rank when it is given its formal name. The basic rank is that of species. The next most important rank is that of genus: when an organism is given a species name it is assigned to a genus, and the genus name is part of the species name. The third-most important rank, although it was not used by Linnaeus, is that of family.

The species name is sometimes called a binomial, that is, a two-term name. For example, the zoological name for the human species is *Homo sapiens*. This is usually italicized in print and underlined when italics are not available. In this case, *Homo* is the generic name and it is capitalized; *sapiens* indicates the species and it is not capitalized.

Ranks in zoology

There are definitions of the following taxonomic ranks in the International Code of Zoological Nomenclature: superfamily, family, subfamily, tribe, subtribe, genus, subgenus, species, subspecies.

The International Code of Zoological Nomenclature divides names into "family-group names", "genus-group names" and "species-group names". The Code explicitly mentions:

Superfamily

Family

Subfamily

Tribe

Subtribe

Genus

Subgenus

Species

Subspecies

The rules in the Code apply to the ranks of superfamily to subspecies, and only to some extent to those above the rank of superfamily. In the "genus group" and "species group" no further ranks are allowed. Among zoologists, additional terms such as *species group*, *species subgroup*, *species complex* and *superspecies* are sometimes used for convenience as extra, but unofficial, ranks between the subgenus and species levels in taxa with many species (e.g., the genus *Drosophila*).

At higher ranks (family and above) a lower level may be denoted by adding the prefix "*infra*", meaning *lower*, to the rank. For example *infra*order (below suborder) or *infra*family (below subfamily).

Names of zoological taxa

- A taxon above the rank of species gets a scientific name in one part (a uninominal name).
- A species gets a name composed of two parts (a binomial name or binomen): generic name + specific name; for example *Canis lupus*.
- A subspecies gets a name composed of three parts (a trinomial name or trinomen): generic name + specific name + subspecific name; for example *Canis lupus familiaris*. As there is only one rank below that of species, no connecting term to indicate rank is used.

Ranks in botany

There are definitions of the following taxonomic ranks in the International Code of Botanical Nomenclature (ICBN): kingdom (regnum), subregnum, division or phylum (divisio, phylum), subdivisio or subphylum, class (classis), subclassis, order (ordo), subordo, family (familia), subfamilia, tribe (tribus), subtribus, genus (genus), subgenus, section (sectio), subsectio, series (series), subseries, species (species), subspecies, variety (varietas), subvarietas, form (forma), subforma.

There are definitions of the following taxonomic ranks in International Code of Nomenclature for Cultivated Plants: cultivar group, cultivar.

According to Art 3.1 of the ICBN the most important ranks of taxa are: kingdom, division or phylum, class, order, family, genus, and species. According to Art 4.1 the secondary ranks of taxa are tribe, section, series, variety and form. There is an indeterminate number of ranks. The ICBN explicitly mentions:

primary ranks

  secondary ranks

    further ranks

kingdom (*regnum*)

    subregnum

division or **phylum** (*divisio, phylum*)

    subdivisio or *subphylum*

class (*classis*)

    subclassis

order (*ordo*)

    subordo

family (*familia*)

    subfamilia

  tribe (*tribus*)

    subtribus

genus (*genus*)

    subgenus

  section (*sectio*)

    subsectio

  series (*series*)

    subseries

species (*species*)

    subspecies

  variety (*varietas*)

    subvarietas

  form (*forma*)

    subforma

The rules in the ICBN apply primarily to the ranks of family and below, and only to some extent to those above the rank of family. Also see descriptive botanical names.

Names of botanical taxa

Of the botanical names used by Linnaeus only names of genera, species and varieties are still used.

Taxa at the rank of genus and above get a botanical name in one part (unitary name); those at the rank of species and above (but below genus) get a botanical name in two parts (binary name); all taxa below the rank of species get a botanical name in three parts (an infraspecific name).

Hybrids can be specified either by a "hybrid formula" that specifies the parentage, or may be given a name. For hybrids getting a hybrid name, the same ranks apply, preceded by "notho", with nothogenus as the highest permitted rank.

Out-dated names for botanical ranks

If a different term for the rank was used in an in old publication, but the intention is clear, botanical nomenclature specifies certain substitutions:

- If names were "intended as names of orders, but published with their rank denoted by a term such as": "cohors" [Latin for "cohort"[3]], "nixus", "alliance", or "Reihe" instead of "order" (Article 17.2), they are treated as names of orders.
- "Family" is substituted for "order" (ordo) or "natural order" (ordo naturalis) under certain conditions where the modern meaning of "order" was not intended. (Article 18.2)
- "Subfamily is substituted for "suborder" (subordo) under certain conditions where the modern meaning of "suborder" was not intended. (Article 19.2)
- In a publication prior to 1 January 1890, if only one infraspecific rank is used, it is considered to be that of variety. (Article 35.4) This commonly applies to publications that labelled infraspecific taxa with Greek letters, α, β, γ, ...

Examples

Classifications of five species follow: the fruit fly so familiar in genetics laboratories (*Drosophila melanogaster*), humans (*Homo sapiens*), the peas used by Gregor Mendel in his discovery of genetics (*Pisum sativum*), the "fly agaric" mushroom *Amanita muscaria*, and the bacterium *Escherichia coli*. The eight major ranks are given in bold; a selection of minor ranks are given as well.

Rank	Fruit fly	Human	Pea	Fly Agaric	*E. coli*
Domain	Eukarya	Eukarya	Eukarya	Eukarya	Bacteria
Kingdom	Animalia	Animalia	Plantae	Fungi	Bacteria
Phylum or **Division**	Arthropoda	Chordata	Magnoliophyta	Basidiomycota	Proteobacteria
Subphylum or subdivision	Hexapoda	Vertebrata	Magnoliophytina	Agaricomycotina	
Class	Insecta	Mammalia	Magnoliopsida	Agaricomycetes	Gammaproteobacteria
Subclass	Pterygota	Theria	Rosidae	Agaricomycetidae	
Order	Diptera	Primates	Fabales	Agaricales	Enterobacteriales
Suborder	Brachycera	Haplorrhini	Fabineae	Agaricineae	
Family	Drosophilidae	Hominidae	Fabaceae	Amanitaceae	Enterobacteriaceae
Subfamily	Drosophilinae	Homininae	Faboideae	Amanitoideae	
Genus	*Drosophila*	*Homo*	*Pisum*	*Amanita*	*Escherichia*

Species	*D. melanogaster*	*H. sapiens*	*P. sativum*	*A. muscaria*	*E. coli*

Table notes

- The ranks of higher taxa, especially intermediate ranks, are prone to revision as new information about relationships is discovered. For example, the traditional classification of primates (class Mammalia — subclass Theria — infraclass Eutheria — order Primates) has been modified by new classifications such as McKenna and Bell (class Mammalia — subclass Theriformes — infraclass Holotheria) with Theria and Eutheria assigned lower ranks between infraclass and the order Primates. See mammal classification for a discussion. These differences arise because there are only a small number of ranks available and a large number of branching points in the fossil record.
- Within species further units may be recognised. Animals may be classified into subspecies (for example, *Homo sapiens sapiens*, modern humans) or morphs (for example *Corvus corax varius* morpha *leucophaeus*, the Pied Raven). Plants may be classified into subspecies (for example, *Pisum sativum* subsp. *sativum*, the garden pea) or varieties (for example, *Pisum sativum* var. *macrocarpon*, snow pea), with cultivated plants getting a cultivar name (for example, *Pisum sativum* var. *macrocarpon* 'Snowbird'). Bacteria may be classified by strains (for example *Escherichia coli* O157:H7, a strain that can cause food poisoning).
- Mnemonics are available at mnemonic-device.eu [4] and thefreedictionary.com [5].

Terminations of names

Taxa above the genus level are often given names based on the type genus, with a standard termination. The terminations used in forming these names depend on the kingdom, and sometimes the phylum and class, as set out in the table below. Pronunciations given are the most Anglicized; more Latinate pronunciations are also common, particularly English pronunciation: /ɑː/ rather than /eɪ/ for stressed *a*.

Rank	Plants	Algae	Fungi	Animals	Bacteria[6]
Division/Phylum	-phyta English pronunciation: /ˈfaɪtə/		-mycota /maɪˈkoʊtə/		
Subdivision/Subphylum	-phytina /fɨˈtaɪnə/		-mycotina /maɪkəˈtaɪnə/		
Class	-opsida /ˈɒpsɨdə/	-phyceae /ˈfaɪʃiː/	-mycetes /maɪˈsiːtiːz/		-ia /iə/
Subclass	-idae /ɨdiː/	-phycidae /ˈfɪsɨdiː/	-mycetidae /maɪˈsɛtɨdiː/		-idae /ɨdiː/
Superorder	-anae /ˈeɪniː/				
Order	-ales /ˈeɪliːz/				-ales /ˈeɪliːz/
Suborder	-ineae /ˈɪnɨ.iː/				-ineae /ˈɪnɨ.iː/
Infraorder	-aria /ˈɛəri.ə/				
Superfamily	-acea /ˈeɪʃə/			-oidea /ˈɔɪdi.ə/	
Epifamily				-oidae /ˈɔɪdiː/	
Family	-aceae /ˈeɪʃiː/			-idae /ɨdiː/	-aceae /ˈeɪʃiː/
Subfamily	-oideae /ˈɔɪdɨ.iː/			-inae /ˈaɪniː/	-oideae /ˈɔɪdɨ.iː/
Infrafamily				-odd /ɒd/[7]	
Tribe	-eae /ɨ.iː/			-ini /ˈaɪnaɪ/	-eae /ɨ.iː/
Subtribe	-inae /ˈaɪniː/			-ina /ˈaɪnə/	-inae /ˈaɪniː/
Infratribe				-ad /æd/	

Table notes

- In botany and mycology names at the rank of family and below are based on the name of a genus, sometimes called the type genus of that taxon, with a standard ending. For example, the rose family Rosaceae is named after the genus *Rosa*, with the standard ending "-aceae" for a family. Names above the rank of family are formed from a family name, or are descriptive (like Gymnospermae or Fungi).
- For animals, there are standard suffixes for taxa only up to the rank of superfamily.[8]
- Forming a name based on a generic name may be not straightforward. For example, the Latin "*homo*" has the genitive "*hominis*", thus the genus "*Homo*" (human) is in the Hominidae, not "Homidae".
- The ranks of epifamily, infrafamily and infratribe (in animals) are used where the complexities of phyletic branching require finer-than-usual distinctions. Although they fall below the rank of superfamily, they are not regulated under the International Code of Zoological Nomenclature and hence do not have formal standard endings. The suffixes listed here are regular, but informal.[9]

All ranks

There is an indeterminate number of ranks, as a taxonomist may invent a new rank at will, at any time, if they feel this is necessary. In doing so, there are some restrictions, which will vary with the nomenclature code which applies.

The following is an artificial synthesis, solely for purposes of demonstration of relative rank (but see notes), from most general to most specific:[10]

- **Domain** *or* **Empire**
  - **Kingdom**
    - Subkingdom
      - Branch
        - Infrakingdom
- Superphylum (*or* Superdivision *in botany*)
  - **Phylum** (*or* **Division** *in botany*)
    - Subphylum (*or* Subdivision *in botany*)
      - Infraphylum (*or* Infradivision *in botany*)
        - Microphylum
- Supercohort (*botany*)[11]
  - Cohort (*botany*)[11]
    - Subcohort (*botany*)[11]
      - Infracohort (*botany*)[11]
- Superclass
  - **Class**
    - Subclass
      - Infraclass
        - Parvclass
- Superdivision (*zoology*)[12]
  - Division (*zoology*)[12]
    - Subdivision (*zoology*)[12]
      - Infradivision (*zoology*)[12]
- Superlegion (*zoology*)
  - Legion (*zoology*)

- Sublegion (*zoology*)
  - Infralegion (*zoology*)
- Supercohort (*zoology*)[11]
  - Cohort (*zoology*)[11]
    - Subcohort (*zoology*)[11]
      - Infracohort (*zoology*)[11]
- Gigaorder (*zoology*)[13]
  - Magnorder *or* Megaorder (*zoology*)[13]
    - Grandorder *or* Capaxorder (*zoology*)[13]
      - Mirorder *or* Hyperorder (*zoology*)[13]
        - Superorder
          - Series (*for fishes*)
            - **Order**
              - Parvorder (*position in some zoological classifications*)
                - Nanorder (*zoology*)
                  - Hypoorder (*zoology*)
                    - Minorder (*zoology*)
                      - Suborder
                        - Infraorder
                          - Parvorder (*usual position*) *or* Microorder (*zoology*)[13]
- Section (*zoology*)
  - Subsection (*zoology*)
- Gigafamily (*zoology*)
  - Megafamily (*zoology*)
    - Grandfamily (*zoology*)
      - Hyperfamily (*zoology*)
        - Superfamily
          - Epifamily (*zoology*)
            - Series (*for Lepidoptera*)
              - Group (*for Lepidoptera*)
                - **Family**
                  - Subfamily
                    - Infrafamily
- Supertribe
  - Tribe
    - Subtribe
      - Infratribe
- **Genus**
  - Subgenus
    - Section (*botany*)

- Subsection (*botany*)
  - Series (*botany*)
    - Subseries (*botany*)
- Superspecies *or* Species-group
  - **Species**
    - Subspecies (*or* Forma Specialis *for fungi, or* Variety *for bacteria*[14])
      - Variety (*botany*) or Form/Morph (*zoology*)
        - Subvariety (*botany*)
          - Form (*botany*)
            - Subform (*botany*)

Significance

Ranks are assigned based on subjective dissimilarity, and do not fully reflect the gradational nature of variation within nature. In most cases, higher taxonomic groupings arise further back in time: not because the rate of diversification was higher in the past, but because each subsequent diversification event results in an increase of diversity and thus increases the taxonomic rank assigned by present-day taxonomists.[15]

Of these many ranks, the most basic is species. However, this is not to say that a taxon at any other rank may not be sharply defined, or that any species is guaranteed to be sharply defined. It varies from case to case. Ideally, nowadays, a taxon is intended to represent a clade, that is, the phylogeny of the organisms under discussion, but this is not a requirement.

See also

- Cladistics

References

[1] International Code of Botanical Nomenclature Online, Vienna Code, 2005, articles 2 and 3 (http://ibot.sav.sk/icbn/main.htm)
[2] International Commission on Zoological Nomenclature (1999) *International Code of Zoological Nomenclature. Fourth Edition.* - International Trust for Zoological Nomenclature, XXIX + 306 pp.
[3] Stearn, W.T. 1992. *Botanical Latin: History, grammar, syntax, terminology and vocabulary, Fourth edition.* David and Charles.
[4] http://www.mnemonic-device.eu/biology
[5] http://acronyms.thefreedictionary.com/KPCOFGS
[6] Bacteriologocal Code (1990 Revision) (http://www.bacterio.cict.fr/classificationgenera.html)
[7] For example, the chelonian infrafamilies Chelodd (Gaffney & Meylan 1988: 169) and Baenodd (*ibid.*, 176).
[8] ICZN article 27.2
[9] As supplied by Gaffney & Meylan (1988).
[10] For the general usage and coordination of zoological ranks between the phylum and family levels, including many intercalary ranks, see Carroll (1988). For additional intercalary ranks in zoology, see especially Gaffney & Meylan (1988); McKenna & Bell (1997); Milner (1988); Novacek (1986, cit. in Carroll 1988: 499, 629); and Paul Sereno's 1986 classification of ornithischian dinosaurs as reported in Lambert (1990: 149, 159). For botanical ranks, including many intercalary ranks, see Willis & McElwain (2002).
[11] In zoological classification, the cohort and its associated group of ranks are inserted between the class group and the ordinal group. In botanical classification, the cohort group has sometimes been inserted between the division (phylum) group and the class group: see Willis & McElwain (2002: 100–101), or has sometimes been used at the rank of order: See International Code of Botanical Nomenclature, Vienna Code 2006, Article 17.2. The cohort has also been used between infraorder and family in saurischian dinosaurs (Benton (http://palaeo.gly.bris.ac.uk/benton/vertclass.html) 2005).
[12] These are movable ranks, most often inserted between the class and the legion or cohort. Nevertheless, their positioning in the zoological hierarchy may be subject to wide variation. For examples, see the Benton classification of vertebrates (http://palaeo.gly.bris.ac.uk/benton/vertclass.html) (2005).
[13] The supra-ordinal sequence gigaorder-megaorder-capaxorder-hyperorder (and the microorder, in roughly the position most often assigned to the parvorder) has been employed in turtles at least (Gaffney & Meylan 1988), while the parallel sequence magnorder-grandorder-mirorder

figures in recently influential classifications of mammals. It is unclear from the sources how these two sequences are to be coordinated (or interwoven) within a unitary zoological hierarchy of ranks. Previously, Novacek (1986) and McKenna-Bell (1997) had inserted mirorders and grandorders between the order and superorder, but Benton (2005) now positions both of these ranks above the superorder.

[14] Additionally, the terms biovar, morphovar and serovar designate bacterial strains (genetic variants) that are physiologically or biochemically distinctive. These are not taxonomic ranks, but are groupings of various sorts which may define a bacterial subspecies.

[15] Error: Bad DOI specified!

Bibliography

- Benton, Michael J. 2005. *Vertebrate Palaeontology*, 3rd ed. Oxford: Blackwell Publishing. ISBN 0-632-05637-1. ISBN 978-0-632-05637-8
- Brummitt, R.K., and C.E. Powell. 1992. *Authors of Plant Names*. Royal Botanic Gardens, Kew. ISBN 0947643443
- Carroll, Robert L. 1988. *Vertebrate Paleontology and Evolution*. New York: W.H. Freeman & Co. ISBN 0-716-7-1822-7
- Gaffney, Eugene S., and Peter A. Meylan. 1988. "A phylogeny of turtles". In M.J. Benton (ed.), *The Phylogeny and Classification of the Tetrapods, Volume 1: Amphibians, Reptiles, Birds*, 157–219. Oxford: Clarendon Press.
- International Association for Plant Taxonomy. 2000. *International Code of Botanical Nomenclature (Saint Louis Code)*, Electronic version. Retrieved on 2007-07-21.
- International Association for Plant Taxonomy. 2006. *International Code of Botanical Nomenclature (Vienna Code)*, Electronic version. Retrieved on 2010-08-19.I (http://ibot.sav.sk/icbn/main.htm)
- Haris Abba Kabara. *Karmos hand book for botanical names*.
- Lambert, David. 1990. *Dinosaur Data Book*. Oxford: Facts On File & British Museum (Natural History). ISBN 0-8160-2431-6
- McKenna, Malcolm C., and Susan K. Bell (editors). 1997. *Classification of Mammals Above the Species Level*. New York: Columbia University Press. ISBN 0-231-11013-8
- Milner, Andrew. 1988. "The relationships and origin of living amphibians". In M.J. Benton (ed.), *The Phylogeny and Classification of the Tetrapods, Volume 1: Amphibians, Reptiles, Birds*, 59–102. Oxford: Clarendon Press.
- Novacek, Michael J. 1986. "The skull of leptictid insectivorans and the higher-level classification of eutherian mammals". *Bulletin of the American Museum of Natural History* **183**: 1–112.
- Sereno, Paul C. 1986. "Phylogeny of the bird-hipped dinosaurs (Order Ornithischia)". *National Geographic Research* **2**: 234–56.
- Willis, K.J., and J.C. McElwain. 2002. *The Evolution of Plants*. Oxford University Press. ISBN 0-19-850065-3

Taxon

A **taxon** (*plural:* **taxa**) is a group of (one or more) organisms, which a taxonomist adjudges to be a unit. Usually a taxon is given a name and a rank, although neither is a requirement. Defining what belongs or does not belong to such a taxonomic group is done by a taxonomist with the science of taxonomy. It is not uncommon for one taxonomist to disagree with another on what exactly belongs to a taxon, or on what exact criteria should be used for inclusion.

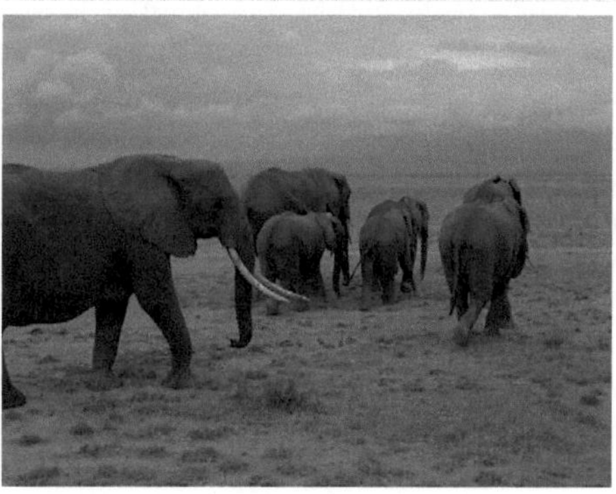
African elephants form a widely-accepted taxon, the genus *Loxodonta*

Taxonomists sometimes make a distinction between "good" (or natural) taxa and others that are "not good" (or artificial). Today it is common to define a good taxon as one that reflects evolutionary (phylogenetic) relationships, but this is not mandatory.

A taxon may be given a formal name, or a scientific name. Such a scientific name is governed by one of the Nomenclature Codes, which sets out rules to determine which scientific name is correct for that particular grouping.

Advocates of phylogenetic nomenclature, using cladistic methods, do require taxa to be monophyletic, consisting of all descendants of some ancestor. They generally do not refer to taxa as their basic unit, but to "clades," a clade being a special form of taxon. However, even in traditional nomenclature, few taxonomists of our time would establish new taxa that they know to be paraphyletic.[1] A famous example of a widely accepted taxon that is not also a clade is the "Reptilia."

Definition

The Glossary of the ***International Code of Zoological Nomenclature*** (1999) defines[2] a

- "taxon, (pl. taxa), n.

> A taxonomic unit, whether named or not: i.e. a population, or group of populations of organisms which are usually inferred to be phylogenetically related and which have characters in common which differentiate (q.v.) the unit (e.g. a geographic population, a genus, a family, an order) from other such units. A taxon encompasses all included taxa of lower rank (q.v.) and individual organisms. [...]"

But there are other definitions.

Ranks

A taxon can be assigned a rank, usually (but not necessarily) when it is given a formal name. The rank of a given taxon is not necessarily fixed, but can be altered later by another (or the same) taxonomist.

"Phylum" applies formally to any biological domain, but traditionally it was always used for animals, whereas "Division" was traditionally often used for plants, fungi, etc.

A prefix is used to indicate a ranking of lesser importance. The prefix *super-* indicates a rank above, the prefix *sub-* indicates a rank below. In zoology the prefix *infra-* indicates a rank below *sub-*. For instance, among the additional ranks of class are superclass, subclass and infraclass.

Rank is relative, and restricted to a particular systematic schema. For example, liverworts have been grouped, in various systems of classification, as a family, order, class, or division (phylum). The use of a narrow set of ranks is challenged by users of cladistics; for example, the mere 10 ranks traditionally used between animal families (governed by the ICZN) and animal phyla (usually the highest relevant rank in taxonomic work) often cannot adequately represent the evolutionary history as more about a lineage's phylogeny becomes known. In addition, the class rank is quite often not an evolutionary but a phenetical and paraphyletic group and as opposed to those ranks governed by the ICZN, can usually not be made monophyletic by exchanging the taxa contained therein. This has given rise to phylogenetic taxonomy and the ongoing development of the *PhyloCode*, which is to govern the application of names to clades.

Life
Domain
Kingdom
Phylum
Class
Order
Family
Genus
Species

The hierarchy of biological classification's eight major taxonomic ranks, which is an example of definition by genus and differentia. Intermediate minor rankings are not shown.

See also

- ABCD Schema
- Alpha taxonomy
- Folk taxonomy
- Chresonym
- Cladistics
- International Code of Botanical Nomenclature (ICBN)
- International Code of Zoological Nomenclature (ICZN)
- Rank (botany)
- Rank (zoology)
- Segregate (taxonomy)

References

[1] de Queiroz, K & J Gauthier (1990). "Phylogeny as a Central Principle in Taxonomy: Phylogenetic Definitions of Taxon Names" (http://vertebrates.si.edu/herps/herps_pdfs/deQueiroz_pdfs/1990deQ_GauSZ.pdf) (PDF). *Systematic Zoology* **39** (4): 307–322. doi:10.2307/2992353. JSTOR 2992353. .

[2] ICZN (1999) International Code of Zoological Nomenclature. Glossary (http://www.iczn.org/iczn/index.jsp?booksection=glossary&nfv=true&mF=). International Commission on Zoological Nomenclature.

Biological_classification

Biological classification, or *scientific classification in biology*, is a method to group and categorize organisms into groups such as genus or species. These groups are known as **taxa** (singular: **taxon**). Biological classification is part of scientific taxonomy.

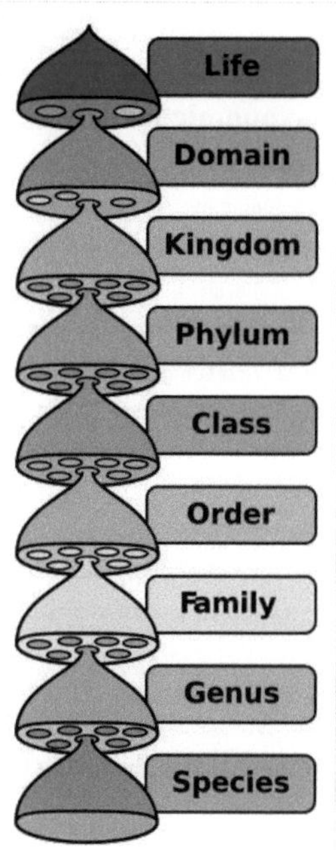

The hierarchy of biological classification's eight major taxonomic ranks, which is an example of definition by genus and differentia. Intermediate minor rankings are not shown.

Modern biological classification has its root in the work of Carolus Linnaeus, who grouped species according to shared physical characteristics. These groupings have since been revised to improve consistency with the Darwinian principle of common descent. With the introduction of the cladistic method in the late 20th century, phylogenetic taxonomy in which organisms are grouped based purely on inferred evolutionary relatedness, ignoring morphological similarity, has become common in some areas of biology.[1] Molecular phylogenetics, which uses DNA sequences as data, has also driven many recent revisions and is likely to continue doing so. Biological classification belongs to the science of biological systematics.

Definition

Classification has been defined by Ernst Mayr as "The arrangement of entities in a hierarchical series of nested classes, in which similar or related classes at one hierarchical level are combined comprehensively into more inclusive classes at the next higher level." A class is defined as "a collection of similar entities".[2] (Note that the word "class" is used quite separately for one of the levels in the biological hierarchy.)

What makes biological classification different from other classification systems (e.g. classifying books in a library) is evolution: the similarity between organisms placed in the same taxon is not arbitrary, but is instead a result of shared descent from their nearest common ancestor. Accordingly, the important attributes or traits for biological classification are 'homologous', i.e., inherited from common ancestors.[3] These must be separated from traits that are analogous. Thus birds and bats both have the power of flight, but this similarity is not used to classify them into a taxon (a "class"), because it is not inherited from a common ancestor. In spite of all the other differences between them, the fact that bats and whales both feed their young on milk is one of the features used to classify both of them as mammals, since it was inherited from a common ancestor(s).

Determining whether similarities are homologous or analogous can be difficult. Thus until recently, golden moles, found in South Africa, were placed in the same taxon (insectivores) as Northern Hemisphere moles, on the basis of morphological and behavioural similarities. However, molecular analysis has shown that they are not closely related, so that their similarities must be due to convergent evolution and not to shared descent, and so should not be used to place them in the same taxon.[4]

Biological types

The scientific names of taxa are formally attached to a **type**, which is one particular specimen (or in some cases a group of specimens, or in some cases an illustration) of the organism, preserved in a museum. The type is the example that serves to anchor or centralize the defining features of each particular taxon.

Taxonomic ranks

A classification as defined above is hierarchical. In a biological classification, **rank** is the level (the relative position) in a hierarchy. (Rarely, the term "taxonomic category" is used instead of "rank".) The *International Code of Zoological Nomenclature* defines rank, in the nomenclatural sense, as:

> The level, for nomenclatural purposes, of a taxon in a taxonomic hierarchy (e.g. all families are for nomenclatural purposes at the same rank, which lies between superfamily and subfamily).[5]

There are seven main ranks defined by the international nomenclature codes: kingdom, phylum/division, class, order, family, genus, species. "Domain", a level above kingdom, has become popular in recent years, but has not been accepted into the codes. Ranks between the seven main ones can be produced by adding prefixes such as "super-", "sub-" or "infra-". Thus a subclass has a rank between class and order, a superfamily between order and family. There are slightly different ranks for zoology and for botany, including subdivisions such as tribe.

Ranks are somewhat arbitrary, but hope to encapsulate the diversity contained within a group — a rough measure of the number of diversifications that the group has been through.[6]

Early systems

Ancient through medieval times

Current systems of classifying forms of life descend from the thought presented by the Greek philosopher Aristotle, who published in his metaphysical works the first known classification of everything whatsoever, or "being". This is the scheme that gave such words as 'substance', 'species' and 'genus' and was retained in modified and less general form by Linnaeus.

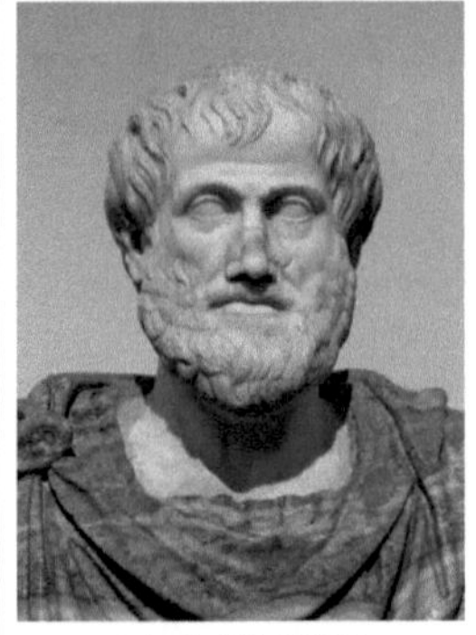

Aristotle, 384–322 BC.

Aristotle also studied animals and classified them according to method of reproduction, as did Linnaeus later with plants. Aristotle's animal classification was eventually made obsolete by additional knowledge and forgotten.

The philosophical classification is in brief as follows:[7] Primary *substance* is the individual being; for example, Peter, Paul, etc. Secondary substance is a predicate that can properly or characteristically be said of a class of primary substances; for example, man of Peter, Paul, etc. The characteristic must not be merely in the individual; for example, being skilled in grammar. Grammatical skill leaves most of Peter out and therefore is not characteristic of him. Similarly man (all of mankind) is not in Peter; rather, he is in man.

Species is the secondary substance that is most proper to its individuals. The most characteristic thing that can be said of Peter is that Peter is a man. An identity is being postulated: "man" is equal to all its individuals and only those individuals. Members of a species differ only in number but are totally the same type.

Genus is a secondary substance less characteristic of and more general than the species; for example, man is an animal, but not all animals are men. It is clear that a genus contains species. There is no limit to the number of Aristotelian genera that might be found to contain the species. Aristotle does not structure the genera into phylum, class, etc., as the Linnaean classification does.

The secondary substance that distinguishes one species from another within a genus is the specific difference. Man can thus be comprehended as the sum of specific differences (the "differentiae" of biology) in less and less general categories. This sum is the definition; for example, man is an animate, sensate, rational substance. The most characteristic definition contains the species and the next most general genus: man is a rational animal. Definition is thus based on the unity problem: the species is but one yet has many differentiae.

The very top genera are the categories. There are ten: one of substance and nine of "accidents", universals that must be "in" a substance. Substances exist by themselves; accidents are only in them: quantity, quality, etc. There is no higher category, "being", because of the following problem, which was only solved in the Middle Ages by Thomas Aquinas: a specific difference is not characteristic of its genus. If man is a rational animal, then rationality is not a property of animals. Substance therefore cannot be a *kind* of being because it can have no specific difference, which would have to be *non*-being.

The problem of "being" occupied the attention of scholastics during the time of the Middle Ages. The solution of St. Thomas, termed the analogy of being, established the field of ontology, which received the better part of the publicity and also drew the line between philosophy and experimental science. The latter rose in the Renaissance from practical technique. Linnaeus, a classical scholar, combined the two on the threshold of the neo-classicist revival now called the Age of Enlightenment.

Renaissance through Age of Reason

An important advance was made by the Swiss professor, Conrad von Gesner (1516–1565). Gesner's work was a critical compilation of life known at the time.

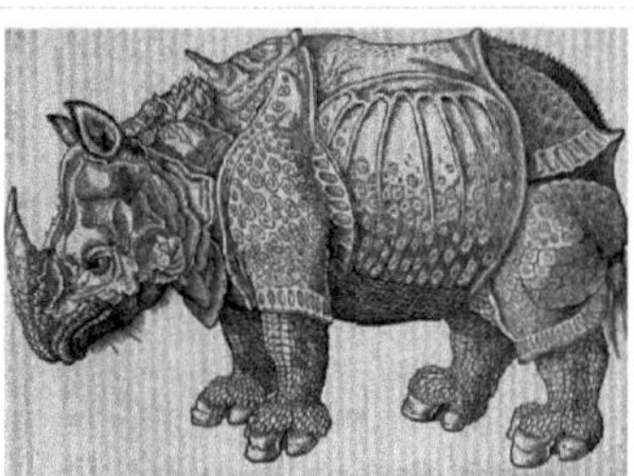

Rhinoceros in Conrad Gesner's *Historiae animalium*, 1551

The exploration of parts of the New World by Europeans produced large numbers of new plants and animals that needed descriptions and classification. The old systems made it difficult to study and locate all these new specimens within a collection and often the same plants or animals were given different names simply because there were too many species to keep track of. A system was needed that could group these specimens together so they could be found; the binomial system was developed based on morphology with groups having similar appearances. In the latter part of the 16th century and the beginning of the 17th, careful study of animals commenced, which, directed first to familiar kinds, was gradually extended until it formed a sufficient body of knowledge to serve as an anatomical basis for classification. Advances in using this knowledge to classify living beings bear a debt to the research of medical anatomists, such as Fabricius (1537–1619), Petrus Severinus (1580–1656), William Harvey (1578–1657), and Edward Tyson (1649–1708). Advances in classification due to the work of entomologists and the first microscopists is due to the research of people like Marcello Malpighi (1628–1694), Jan Swammerdam (1637–1680), and Robert Hooke (1635–1702). Lord Monboddo (1714–1799) was one of the early abstract thinkers whose works illustrate knowledge of species relationships and who foreshadowed the theory of evolution.[8]

Early methodists

Since late in the 15th century, a number of authors had become concerned with what they called *methodus,* (method). By method authors mean an arrangement of minerals, plants, and animals according to the principles of logical division. The term *Methodists* was coined by Carolus Linnaeus in his *Bibliotheca Botanica* to denote the authors who care about the principles of classification (in contrast to the mere *collectors* who are concerned primarily with the description of plants paying little or no attention to their arrangement into genera, etc.). Important early Methodists were Italian philosopher, physician, and botanist Andrea Caesalpino, English naturalist John Ray, German physician and botanist Augustus Quirinus Rivinus, and French physician, botanist, and traveller Joseph Pitton de Tournefort.

Andrea Caesalpino (1519–1603) in his *De plantis libri XVI* (1583) proposed the first methodical arrangement of plants. On the basis of the structure of trunk and fructification he divided plants into fifteen "higher genera".

John Ray (1627–1705) was an English naturalist who published important works on plants, animals, and natural theology. The approach he took to the classification of plants in his Historia Plantarum was an important step towards modern taxonomy. Ray rejected the system of dichotomous division by which species were classified according to a pre-conceived, either/or type system, and instead classified plants according to similarities and differences that emerged from observation.

Both Caesalpino and Ray used traditional plant names and thus, the name of a plant did not reflect its taxonomic position (e.g. even though the apple and the peach belonged to different "higher genera" of John Ray's *methodus*, both retained their traditional names *Malus* and *Malus Persica* respectively). A further step was taken by Rivinus and Pitton de Tournefort who made genus a distinct rank within taxonomic hierarchy and introduced the practice of naming the plants according to their genera.

Augustus Quirinus Rivinus (1652–1723), in his classification of plants based on the characters of the flower, introduced the category of order (corresponding to the "higher" genera of John Ray and Andrea Caesalpino). He was the first to abolish the ancient division of plants into herbs and trees and insisted that the true method of division should be based on the parts of the fructification alone. Rivinus extensively used dichotomous keys to define both orders and genera. His method of naming plant species resembled that of Joseph Pitton de Tournefort. The names of all plants belonging to the same genus should begin with the same word (generic name). In the genera containing more than one species the first species was named with generic name only, while the second, etc. were named with a combination of the generic name and a modifier (*differentia specifica*).

Joseph Pitton de Tournefort (1656–1708) introduced an even more sophisticated hierarchy of class, section, genus, and species. He was the first to use consistently the uniformly composed species names that consisted of a generic name and a many-worded diagnostic phrase *differentia specifica.* Unlike Rivinus, he used *differentiae* with all species of polytypic genera.

Linnaean taxonomy

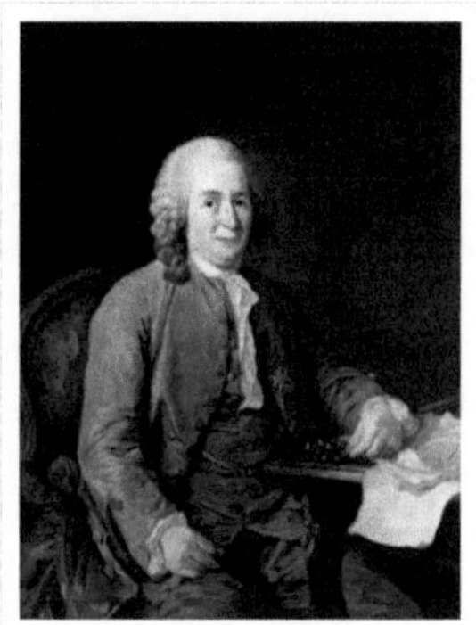

Carolus Linnaeus

Carolus Linnaeus' great work, the *Systema Naturæ* (1st ed. 1735), ran through twelve editions during his lifetime. In this work, nature was divided into three kingdoms: mineral, vegetable and animal. Linnaeus used five ranks: class, order, genus, species, and variety.

He abandoned long descriptive names of classes and orders still used by his immediate predecessors (Rivinus and Pitton de Tournefort) and replaced them with single-word names, provided genera with detailed diagnoses (*characteres naturales*), and combined numerous varieties into their species, thus saving botany from the chaos of new forms produced by horticulturalists.

Linnaeus is best known for his introduction of the method still used to formulate the scientific name of every species. Before Linnaeus, long many-worded names (composed of a generic name and a *differentia specifica*) had been used, but as these names gave a description of the species, they were not fixed. In his *Philosophia Botanica* (1751) Linnaeus took every effort to improve the composition and reduce the length of the many-worded names by abolishing unnecessary rhetorics, introducing new descriptive terms and defining their meaning with an unprecedented precision. In the late 1740s Linnaeus began to use a parallel system of naming species with *nomina trivialia. Nomen triviale*, a trivial name, was a single- or two-word epithet placed on the margin of the page next to the many-worded "scientific" name. The only rules Linnaeus applied to them was that the trivial names should be short, unique within a given genus, and that they should not be changed. Linnaeus consistently applied *nomina trivialia* to the species of plants in *Species Plantarum* (1st edn. 1753) and to the species of animals in the 10th edition of *Systema Naturæ* (1758).

By consistently using these specific epithets, Linnaeus separated nomenclature from description. Even though the parallel use of *nomina trivialia* and many-worded descriptive names continued until late in the eighteenth century, it was gradually replaced by the practice of using shorter proper names consisting of the generic name and the trivial name of the species. In the nineteenth century, this new practice was codified in the first Rules and Laws of Nomenclature, and the 1st edn. of *Species Plantarum* and the 10th edn. of *Systema Naturae* were chosen as starting points for the Botanical and Zoological Nomenclature respectively. This convention for naming species is referred to as binomial nomenclature.

Today, nomenclature is regulated by Nomenclature Codes, which allows names divided into taxonomic ranks.

Modern system

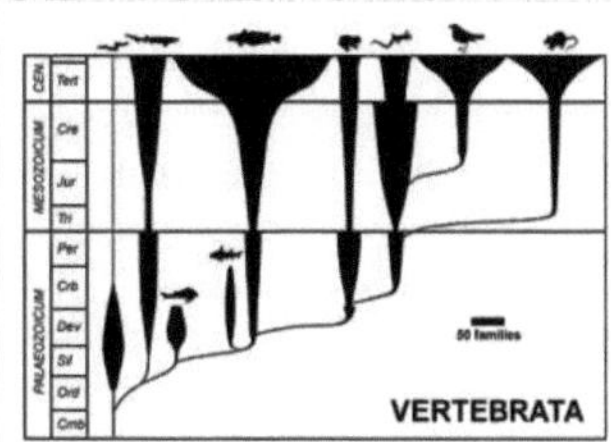

Evolution of the vertebrates at class level, width of spindles indicating number of families. Spindle diagrams are typical for Evolutionary taxonomy

Whereas Linnaeus classified for ease of identification, the idea of the Linnaean taxonomy as translating into a sort of dendrogram of the Animal- and Plant Kingdoms was formulated toward the end of the 18th century, well before the *On the Origin of Species* was published. Among early works exploring the idea of a transmutation of species was Erasmus Darwin's 1796 Zoönomia and Jean-Baptiste Lamarck's Philosophie Zoologique of 1809. The idea was popularised in the Anglophone world by the speculative, but widely read Vestiges of the Natural History of Creation, published anonymously by Robert Chambers in 1844.[9]

With Darwin's theory, a general acceptance that classification should reflect the Darwinian principle of common descent quickly appeared. Tree of Life representations became popular in scientific works, with known fossil groups incorporated. One of the first modern groups tied to fossil ancestors were birds. Using the then newly discovered fossils of *Archaeopteryx* and *Hesperornis*, Thomas Henry Huxley pronounced that they had evolved from dinosaurs, a group formally named by Richard Owen in 1842.[10] The resulting description, that of dinosaurs "giving rise to" or being "the ancestors of" birds, is the essential hallmark of evolutionary taxonomic thinking. As more and more fossil groups were found and recognized in the late 19th and early 20th century, palaeontologists worked to understand the history of animals through the ages by linking together known groups[11] With the modern evolutionary synthesis of the early 1940s, an essentially modern understanding of evolution of the major groups was in place. The evolutionary taxonomy being based on Linnaean taxonomic ranks, the two terms are largely interchangeable in modern use.

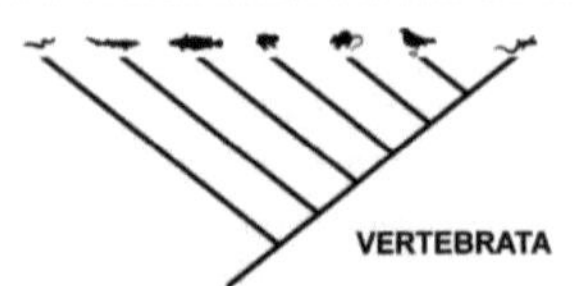

The same relationship, expressed as a cladogram typical for cladistics

Since the 1960s a trend called phylogenetic nomenclature (or cladism) has emerged, inspired by the cladistic method. The salient feature is arranging taxa in a hierarchical evolutionary tree, ignoring ranks. If a taxon includes all the descendants of some ancestral form, it is called monophyletic. Groups that have descendant groups removed from them (e.g. dinosaurs, with birds as offspring group) are termed paraphyletic, while groups representing more than one branch from the tree of life are called polyphyletic. A formal code of nomenclature, the *International Code of Phylogenetic Nomenclature*, or *PhyloCode* for short, is currently under development, intended to deal with names of clades. Linnaean ranks will be optional under the *PhyloCode*, which is intended to coexist with the current, rank-based codes.

Kingdoms and domains

From well before Linnaeus, plants and animals were considered separate Kingdoms. Linnaeus used this as the top rank, dividing the physical world into the plant, animal and mineral kingdoms. As advances in microscopy made classification of microorganisms possible, the number of kingdoms increased, five and six-kingdom systems being the most common.

Domains are a relatively new grouping. The three-domain system was first proposed in 1990, but not generally accepted until later. One main characteristic of the three-domain method is the separation of Archaea and Bacteria, previously grouped into the single kingdom Bacteria (a kingdom also sometimes called Monera). Consequently, the three domains of life are conceptualized as Archaea, Bacteria, and Eukaryota (comprising the nuclei-bearing eukaryotes).[12] A small minority of scientists add Archaea as a sixth kingdom, but do not accept the domain method.

Thomas Cavalier-Smith, who has published extensively on the classification of protists, has recently proposed that the Neomura, the clade that groups together the Archaea and Eukarya, would have evolved from Bacteria, more precisely from Actinobacteria. His classification of 2004 treats the archaebacteria as part of a subkingdom of the Kingdom Bacteria, i.e. he rejects the three-domain system entirely.[13]

Linnaeus 1735[14] 2 kingdoms	Haeckel 1866[15] 3 kingdoms	Chatton 1925[16] [17] 2 empires	Copeland 1938[18] [19] 4 kingdoms	Whittaker 1969[20] 5 kingdoms	Woese et al. 1977[21] [22] 6 kingdoms	Woese et al. 1990[23] 3 domains	Cavalier-Smith 2004[13] 6 kingdoms
(not treated)	Protista	Prokaryota	Monera	Monera	Eubacteria	Bacteria	Bacteria
					Archaebacteria	Archaea	
		Eukaryota	Protoctista	Protista	Protista	Eukarya	Protozoa
							Chromista
Vegetabilia	Plantae		Plantae	Plantae	Plantae		Plantae
			Protoctista	Fungi	Fungi		Fungi
Animalia	Animalia		Animalia	Animalia	Animalia		Animalia

Authorities (author citation)

An "authority" may be placed after a scientific name. The authority is the name of the scientist who first validly published the name. For example, in 1758 Linnaeus gave the Asian elephant the scientific name *Elephas maximus*, so the name is sometimes written as "*Elephas maximus* Linnaeus, 1758". The names of authors are frequently abbreviated: the abbreviation "L." is universally accepted for Linnaeus, and in botany there is a regulated list of standard abbreviations (see list of botanists by author abbreviation). The system for assigning authorities differs slightly between botany and zoology. However, it is standard that if a species' name or placement has been changed since the original description, the original authority's name is placed in parentheses.

Globally unique identifiers for names

There is a movement within the biodiversity informatics community to provide globally unique identifiers in the form of Life Science Identifiers (LSID) for all biological names. This would allow authors to cite names unambiguously in electronic media and reduce the significance of errors in the spelling of names or the abbreviation of authority names. Three large nomenclatural databases (referred to as nomenclators) have already begun this process, these are Index Fungorum, International Plant Names Index and ZooBank. Other databases, that publish taxonomic rather than nomenclatural data, have also started using LSIDs to identify **taxa**. The key example of this is Catalogue of Life. In the next step in integration, these taxonomic databases will include references to the nomenclatural databases using LSIDs.

See also

- All Species Foundation
- Holotype
- International Code of Nomenclature for algae, fungi, and plants
- International Code of Zoological Nomenclature
- List of Latin and Greek words commonly used in systematic names
- Phenetics
- Phylogenetic tree
- Species description
- Tree of Life Web Project
- Trinomial nomenclature
- Type (biology)

- Virus classification

References

[1] Laurin, M. (2010). "The subjective nature of Linnaean categories and its impact in evolutionary biology and biodiversity studies" (http://www.ctoz.nl/ctz/vol79/nr04/art01). *Contributions to Zoology* **79** (4). . Retrieved 21 March 2012.

[2] Mayr, Ernst & Bock, W.J. (2002). "Classifications and other ordering systems". *J. Zool. Syst. Evol. Research* **40** (4): 169–94. doi:10.1046/j.1439-0469.2002.00211.x.

[3] Mayr & Bock 2002, p. 178

[4] Mayr & Bock 2002, p. 178ff

[5] International Commission on Zoological Nomenclature (1999) *International Code of Zoological Nomenclature. Fourth Edition.* - International Trust for Zoological Nomenclature, XXIX + 306 pp.

[6] Error: Bad DOI specified!

[7] *Categories* Section 5 and *Metaphysics* Book 6, but the terms are used in many places throughout the writings of Aristotle.

[8] "Nomina Circumscribentia Insectorum" (http://www.insecta.bio.pu.ru). . Retrieved 2008-10-09.

[9] Secord, James A. (2000). *Victorian Sensation: The Extraordinary Publication, Reception, and Secret Authorship of Vestiges of the Natural History of Creation* (http://www.press.uchicago.edu/cgi-bin/hfs.cgi/00/14098.ctl). Chicago: University of Chicago Press. ISBN 978-0-226-74410-0. .

[10] Huxley, T.H. (1876): Lectures on Evolution. *New York Tribune*. Extra. no 36. In Collected Essays IV: pp 46-138 original text w/ figures (http://aleph0.clarku.edu/huxley/CE4/LecEvol.html)

[11] Rudwick, M. J. S. (1985). *The Meaning of Fossils: Episodes in the History of Palaeontology*. University of Chicago Press. p. 24. ISBN 0226731030

[12] See especially pp. 45, 78 and 555 of Joel Cracraft and Michael J. Donaghue, eds. (2004). *Assembling the Tree of Life*. Oxford, England: Oxford University Press.

[13] Cavalier-Smith, T. (2004), "Only six kingdoms of life" (http://www.cladocera.de/protozoa/cavalier-smith_2004_prs.pdf), *Proc. R. Soc. Lond. B* **271**: 1251–62, doi:10.1098/rspb.2004.2705, PMC 1691724, PMID 15306349, , retrieved 2010-04-29

[14] C. Linnaeus (1735). *Systemae Naturae, sive regna tria naturae, systematics proposita per classes, ordines, genera & species.*

[15] E. Haeckel (1866). *Generelle Morphologie der Organismen*. Reimer, Berlin.

[16] É. Chatton (1925). "*Pansporella perplexa*. Réflexions sur la biologie et la phylogénie des protozoaires". *Ann. Sci. Nat. Zool* **10-VII**: 1–84.

[17] É. Chatton (1937). *Titres et Travaux Scientifiques (1906–1937)*. Sette, Sottano, Italy.

[18] H. Copeland (1938). "The kingdoms of organisms". *Quarterly Review of Biology* **13**: 383–420. doi:10.1086/394568.

[19] H. F. Copeland (1956). *The Classification of Lower Organisms*. Palo Alto: Pacific Books.

[20] Whittaker RH (January 1969). "New concepts of kingdoms of organisms". *Science* **163** (3863): 150–60. doi:10.1126/science.163.3863.150. PMID 5762760.

[21] C. R. Woese, W. E. Balch, L. J. Magrum, G. E. Fox and R. S. Wolfe (August 1977). "An ancient divergence among the bacteria". *Journal of Molecular Evolution* **9** (4): 305–311. doi:10.1007/BF01796092. PMID 408502.

[22] Woese CR, Fox GE (November 1977). "Phylogenetic structure of the prokaryotic domain: the primary kingdoms". *Proc. Natl. Acad. Sci. U.S.A.* **74** (11): 5088–90. doi:10.1073/pnas.74.11.5088. PMC 432104. PMID 270744.

[23] Woese C, Kandler O, Wheelis M (1990). "Towards a natural system of organisms: proposal for the domains Archaea, Bacteria, and Eucarya." (http://www.pnas.org/cgi/reprint/87/12/4576). *Proc Natl Acad Sci U S A* **87** (12): 4576–9. Bibcode 1990PNAS...87.4576W. doi:10.1073/pnas.87.12.4576. PMC 54159. PMID 2112744. .

Bibliography

- Atran, S. (1990). *Cognitive foundations of natural history: towards an anthropology of science*. Cambridge, England: Cambridge University Press. xii+360 pages. ISBN 0521372933, 0521372933.
- Larson, J. L. (1971). *Reason and experience. The representation of Natural Order in the work of Carl von Linne.* Berkeley, California: University of California Press. VII+171 pages.
- Mayr, Ernst & Bock, W.J. (2002). "Classifications and other ordering systems". *J. Zool. Syst. Evol. Research* **40** (4): 169–94. doi:10.1046/j.1439-0469.2002.00211.x.
- Schuh, R. T. and A. V. Z. Brower. (2009). *Biological Systematics: principles and applications (2nd edn.)* Cornell University Press xiii+311 pages. ISBN 978-0-8014-4799-0
- Species 2000 & ITIS Catalogue of Life 2008 (http://www.catalogueoflife.org/annual-checklist/2008/browse_taxa.php)
- Stafleau, F. A. (1971). *Linnaeus and the Linnaeans. The spreading of their ideas in systematic botany, 1753–1789*. Utrecht: Oosthoek. xvi+386 pages.

Article Sources and Contributors

Family_(biology) *Source*: http://en.wikipedia.org/w/index.php?title=Family_%28biology%29 *Contributors*: A8UDI, AdjustShift, Aezram, Aitias, Alansohn, Alexei Kouprianov, Alfio, Andonic, Andre Engels, AndrewWTaylor, Andyjsmith, AnonymousHaxker, Avoided, Awesomefuture, BD2412, Baschi Moleski, BengMog, Bhinsee, Binwindinshin, Bogey97, Bootstoots, Brya, Bryan Derksen, Butwhatdoiknow, CRICKETLtd, CZmarlin, CanadianLinuxUser, Captain-tucker, Cburnett, Cforrester101, DWeir, Dalt54321, Dave6, Delldot, Dendrid, DerHexer, Dougweller, Drmies, ENeville, ESkog, Eatoncheese, El C, Elassint, En-Cu-Kou, Erdigenc, Fabartus, Falcon8765, Farosdaughter, Flewis, Fluffernutter, Fram, FredMSloniker, Fresh dog, Frogthedog, Garry192837, Gary King, Geniac, Glenn, Gnostrat, Gribskov, Gromlakh, Gunnar Hendrich, Gökhan, Hatmatbbat10, Hayabusa future, IEatToothpaste, Invertzoo, ItsZippy, J.delanoy, J36miles, JaGa, Japanese Searobin, Jauhienij, Josh Grosse, Jrockley, Kahkonen, Katimawan2005, KevinHanshiWu2, Kgn sm, L Kensington, Lanareader6, Levineps, LiDaobing, Lightmouse, Logan, Lolbuddy1997, Look2See1, Lucyin, MC10, MPF, Magnus Manske, Malik Shabazz, Matthew.danaher.12, Merope, Mgiganteus1, MiShogun, Multichill, Neelix, Nihiltres, Nik42, Node ue, Numbo3, Oxymoron83, PamD, Pax:Vobiscum, Pbj123, Philip Trueman, PierreAbbat, Pinethicket, Pingveno, Pippu d'Angelo, Pseudomonas, Ram-Man, Randigrace, Rjwilmsi, Romanskolduns, Rugbyboyrob, SMP, SarahMuffin, SatuSuro, Sheep81, Shuipzv3, Siim, Silence, Smith609, Snek01, Snowmanradio, Sopoforic, Soumyasch, SpyMagician, Sreejithk2000, Standproud1, Stemonitis, Stevenmitchell, Synchronism, TWCarlson, TangoFett, Tannin, Tempodivalse, Tommy2010, Tompw, Tstormcandy, Ulric1313, Victor falk, Vuong Ngan Ha, W4chris, Wideshanks, WikHead, WikiPuppies, Wikid77, Wikitanvir, William Avery, WolfmanSF, Xxxxlällällällä, Yerpo, Yosri, Zachary, 207 anonymous edits

Protein_subfamily *Source*: http://en.wikipedia.org/w/index.php?title=Protein_subfamily *Contributors*: D6, DuncanHill, Groiby, JaGa, Jessemv, Jongbhak, Kkmurray, Malcolma, Nima1024, Tikojan, Ziounclesi, 3 anonymous edits

Phylum *Source*: http://en.wikipedia.org/w/index.php?title=Phylum *Contributors*: 100110100, 2004-12-29T22:45Z, 28421u2232nfenfcenc, ABXDataLogic, Abrech, Agk1998, Alan Liefting, Alansohn, Alefbe, Alexei Kouprianov, Aljullu, Anomalocaris, Antandrus, Art LaPella, Artman40, Atelaes, Avillia, Avoided, Axlrosen, BD2412, Bejnar, Biermeister, Big Brother 1984, Bigguy12, Bluerasberry, Bobo192, Bongwarrior, BorgQueen, Brandon5485, Branka France, Brendabr, Brya, Bryan Derksen, Butwhatdoiknow, CDN99, Calvin 1998, CanadianLinuxUser, CardinalDan, Cheers!, Choij, Cholerashot, Connormah, Coppertwig, Cristyal1, Crustaceanguy, Csigabi, Cxz111, Dainis, Dana boomer, Danger, Dawd, DerHexer, DewiMorgan, Dizanl, DopefishJustin, EamonnPKeane, El C, Eleven even, Elucidate, EncycloPetey, Eog1916, Epbr123, Eras-mus, Euryalus, Everyking, ExNihilo, Failure.exe, Faradayplank, FisherQueen, Fred Bauder, FreplySpang, Galoubet, Gdr, Gerbrant, Gilliam, Glane23, Gnostrat, Goatasaur, Golgofrinchian, Grendelkhan, Gurch, HJ Mitchell, Haleyga, Hans Dunkelberg, Hgrobe, Hibernian, Honking Antelope, Hordaland, Huttarl, Hveziris, Iapetus, Icairns, ImUrCaptain, Immunize, Iph, Jack Brooks, Jackol, Jacky.cheOng, Jebus989, Jeffrey Mall, Jj137, Jklumker, Jncraton, JohnOwens, Jojhutton, Jon186, Josh Grosse, Jrockley, Kaimiddleton, Kalathalan, Karmosin, Kateshortforbob, Katimawan2005, Keenan Pepper, Keithonearth, Kevin, Khoikhoi, Kidd Loris, KimvdLinde, King of Hearts, Kjaer, Kmw2700, Kolbasz, Koryakov Yuri, KramarDanIkabu, LOL, Labellerien, Lavateraguy, Le temps perdu, Leafeater, LedgendGamer, LegitimateAndEvenCompelling, Lerdsuwa, Leszek Jańczuk, Lisatwo, Lolmaster, Look2See1, Lowellian, Lozeldafan, MER-C, Macedonian, Magioladitis, Mandarax, Manderson198, MathMan64, Mav, Meteor2017, MikeLynch, Mikespedia, Mini-Geek, Mr0t1633, Msheskin, MuZemike, Natalie Erin, NawlinWiki, Ncapriola, Nephtes, Neverquick, NewEnglandYankee, Newone, Niffux, Nihiltres, Nik42, Nivix, Noctibus, Node ue, Obli, Ocaasi, Omnipaedista, Opie, Ordinary Person, Ospalh, OverlordQ, Penhollow, Peter Isotalo, Peter coxhead, Petter Bøckman, Pgan002, Philip Trueman, Pinethicket, Piotrus, Pippu d'Angelo, Plantsurfer, Pmronchi, Prosfilaes, Pseudofusulina, Quietust, R. fiend, RadioFan, Razorflame, Remember the dot, Rjwilmsi, Robert Brockway, Rodasmith, Ronhjones, RoyBoy, Ruduger, Ryan Norton, Salvor, Samak47, Samtheboy, SimonP, Sintaku, Sionnach1, Slon02, Smith609, Smithfarm, Snek01, Some jerk on the Internet, Someguy1221, Sonez1113, Sophie means wisdom, SpaceFlight89, Squidonius, Sssprkrao, StAkAr Karnak, Standproud1, Stemonitis, Stephenb, Steve Newport, SupernovaExplosion, Svick, Synchronism, Syp, Tabletop, Taka, Taterpal, TexasAndroid, The High Fin Sperm Whale, The Thing That Should Not Be, TheLimbicOne, Thecheesykid, Thegargoylevine, Tide rolls, Tideflat, Tiffers1441, Timwi, Tommy2010, Tompw, TowTrucker, Treworman, TripleAven, Ulric1313, Unfree, Ute in DC, Vanished User 1004, Vanished User 4517, Victor falk, Vinsfan368, Vojtech.dostal, Vsmith, Vuong Ngan Ha, Vuongc, Wackywace, Wayne Slam, Welsh, Wes!, Westandrew.g, Wetman, Whkoh, WikiLolz001, Wikiborg, Wikipelli, William Avery, Willking1979, Wknight94, WolfmanSF, Wtmitchell, XJamRastafire, Xeno, Yamaguchi, Ybk33, Yetisyny, Youyobro, Yuugian, 495 anonymous edits

Class_(biology) *Source*: http://en.wikipedia.org/w/index.php?title=Class_%28biology%29 *Contributors*: Alefbe, Alexei Kouprianov, Amit6, Antzervos, Apokryltaros, Ark-pl, Aruton, AvicAWB, Blablaboo, Brya, Bryan Derksen, Caltas, Christopher1991, Closedmouth, Cremepuff222, DQJK2000, Dcirovic, DeadEyeArrow, Dendrid, DocWatson42, Dogman15, Dorftrottel, E2e3v6, Eifachoeppis, El C, Eog1916, Ettrig, Eugene van der Pijll, Eyeofhorace, FrozenPurpleCube, Fæ, Ginsengbomb, Glenn, Grisunge, J.delanoy, Jason.grossman, Jauhienij, Jay-Sebastos, Jerry Zhang, Jim1138, Jose77, Josh Grosse, Jrockley, Katimawan2005, Kesal, Kevin6025, Kupirijo, Larsroe, Lavateraguy, LedgendGamer, Levineps, Logan, Look2See1, Lurker, MPF, Mav, Mentifisto, MichaK, MrCEO, NatureA16, Nihiltres, Node ue, Opie, Pharaoh of the Wizards, Pippu d'Angelo, Poeloq, Ram-Man, Rjwilmsi, Rockfang, Romanskolduns, Sinn, Smith609, Snek01, Spambit, Standproud1, Tannin, The sock that should not be, Tompw, Tomtom547, Txomin, Victor falk, Vuong Ngan Ha, Werothegreat, White Shadows, Wiki wiki1, WolfmanSF, Xyzzyplugh, Yerpo, 115 anonymous edits

Order_(biology) *Source*: http://en.wikipedia.org/w/index.php?title=Order_%28biology%29 *Contributors*: 1966batfan, 28421u2232nfenfcenc, Aboctok, Aesopos, Alexei Kouprianov, Alfio, Andyjsmith, Antandrus, Apokryltaros, Ballista, Beano, Bento00, BjankuloskiO6en, Bobo192, Brya, Bryan Derksen, CanadianLinuxUser, Chairman S., Coccyx Bloccyx, Dawn Bard, Dendrid, EdBever, EdwardLane, El C, Elipongo, Erdigenc, Ettrig, Eugene van der Pijll, Facugaich, Fama Clamosa, Geoffr, Glenn, Gnostrat, Graham87, Green caterpillar, Grisunge, Gruzd, IvanLanin, Jackol, Jerry Zhang, John, Jonkerz, Jose77, Josh Grosse, Jrockley, Jóna Þórunn, Kappa, Keegscee, KhAnubis, Kimse, Kmoksy, KnowledgeOfSelf, Kostisl, La Pianista, Lavateraguy, Legotech, Lesclaypool397, Lightmouse, Lloydpick, Look2See1, MPF, Magnus Manske, MathMan64, Mav, MiShogun, MichaK, Michaelzeng7, Mike Rosoft, Monk of the highest order, Moonriddengirl, Nihiltres, Node ue, Opie, Orlandomachado, Pb30, Peter coxhead, Pippu d'Angelo, Proski, Protonk, Quartermaster, Ram-Man, Rich Farmbrough, Rjwilmsi, Robofish, SP-KP, Saros136, Seraphim, Shapeev, Silence, Smekh, Smith609, Snek01, Snowmanradio, Standproud1, Stemonitis, Sualah, Summer Song, THEN WHO WAS PHONE?, Tannin, Tombomp, Tompw, Turtleman69545, Unyoyega, Vanished User 4517, Victor falk, Vuong Ngan Ha, WadeSimMiser, Washburnmav, Wikid77, Wimt, Wlodzimierz, WolfmanSF, Ybk33, Ævar Arnfjörð Bjarmason, ملاي, தகவலாழவன், 140 anonymous edits

Genus *Source*: http://en.wikipedia.org/w/index.php?title=Genus *Contributors*: 16@r, 22vampsrock22, 5 albert square, 618116yfp, Abanima, Aitias, Ajraddatz, Alansohn, Alex.muller, Alexei Kouprianov, AlexiusHoratius, Andre Engels, AndrewWTaylor, AnonMoos, Anonymous Dissident, Anthony Appleyard, Aranea Mortem, Arichnad, Art LaPella, AstroNomer, Athaler, AugPi, Austro, Autonova, AxelBoldt, Baranxtu, Belfry, Benjamnjoel2, Berria, Berserkerz Crit, Berton, Betterusername, BjankuloskiO6en, Bobblewik, Bobo192, Bongwarrior, Brian0918, Brianga, Brya, Bryan Derksen, Byron755, CWY2190, Cburnett, Christiangrann, Circeus, CrazyUkee, Cxz111, DMacks, Damnreds, Darth Panda, Daviddariusbijan, Dendrid, DerHexer, Don2k11, Dr CyCoe, Drew roy, Drmies, Dysmorodrepanis, ENeville, ERcheck, ESkog, El C, Eloquence, Emmal700, Enigmaman, Eog1916, Epbr123, Erebus Morgaine, Escape Orbit, Ethien, Firsfron, Flewis, Flyset, Frankenpuppy, Fred Bauder, FreplySpang, FrozenPurpleCube, GB fan, GKoUtSo201, Galoubet, Gdr, GerardM, Giftlite, Gilliam, Gk007, Glacialfox, Glenn, GoEThe, GrahamBould, Graminophile, Grendelkhan, Grunny, Gwern, GüegüeügeMoiraMoira, Hallows AG, Hamamelis, Harloshaply, Hayabusa future, Hbent, Heracles31, Hozro, Hyacinth, I got fived!, Ian Dalziel, Ian.thomson, Icairns, Ignitus, Iliketochangearticles, Innotata, Invertzoo, Iridescent, J.delanoy, JHolman, Jackfork, Jackjackjr, Japanese Searobin, JemGage, Jerzy, Jfioeawfjdls453, Jim1138, Joblax, John KB, John Price, Joseph Solis in Australia, Jossi, Jrockley, Julesd, Julian Mendez, JustAGal, Katimawan2005, Kazenteshi, Kchishol1970, Keilana, KeithTyler, Kesuari, Kimse, Kintaro, Kironide, Kjkolb, Kmsiever, Knutux, Komododragonfan16, Kubigula, Kukini, Kungfuadam, LOL, Lankiveil, Lantianer, Lerdsuwa, Lightmouse, Look2See1, Luckas Blade, Lucyin, MER-C, ML5, MPF, MWAK, Macedonian, Madhero88, Maelin, Maildej, Mani1, Marek69, Maristoddard, Marshman, MartinezMD, Mauler90, Mav, Merovingian, Meteor2017, MezzoDragon, Mfwitten, Mgiganteus1, MichaelSeemann, Mikael Häggström, Mike Dillon, Mike Searson, Mikepenny01, MisfitToys, Mjster, Mmcknight4, Ms2ger, Muhaha, Mukkakukaku, Nakon, NewEnglandYankee, Nihiltres, Nivlak, Nnof002, Nsaa, Nutzmonkey, Oneiros, Orphan Wiki, Pageleft, Paul August, Paul-L, Pengo, Philip Trueman, PierreAbbat, Pinethicket, Pippu d'Angelo, Prashant.saxena, R.e.b., Ram-Man, RazorICE, Redaktor, RexNL, Rich Farmbrough, Richard New Forest, Richard0715, Rid9, Rjwilmsi, Robert Foley, RobertG, Romanskolduns, Ronhjones, Rossco89, RoundAbout949, Rvollmert, S3000, SP-KP, Salamurai, Sarahcwilkins, Satellite9876, Scientizzle, Sciurinæ, Seahorseruler, Shirt58, Shulei-shulei, SimonP, Sluzzelin, Smith609, Snek01, Snowmanradio, Spiff, Srios653, Standproud1, Starks, Stemonitis, Sumansetty, Super Mario, Taztouzi1, The Earwig, The Final Chronicler, Tide rolls, Tobias Bergemann, Tommy2010, TotoBaggins, Unara, Uncle G, Unyoyega, Uscumow17, UtherSRG, Velho, Verbum Veritas, Victor falk, Vietbio, Vina, Vishnava, Vsmith, Wavelength, We.eter, Werts335, Whosyourjudas, Wilbozz, Williamb, Wisco, WolfmanSF, YellowMonkey, Yerpo, Yonwe, Yosri, YuKornilev, Zumbo, Саша Стефановић, 372 anonymous edits

Species *Source*: http://en.wikipedia.org/w/index.php?title=Species *Contributors*: ...hellohere..*, 132.235.232.xxx, 165.123.179.xxx, 19.168, 192.18.98.xxx, 2004-12-29T22:45Z, 4twenty42o, 5 albert square, AC+79 3888, Abbeyvet, Abdullais4u, Abyssal, Access Denied, Acer123456, Adam1213, Addshore, Adzyaye, Aervanath, Ahoerstemeier, Aircorn, AlanBarrett, Alanl, Alansohn, Aldaniel, Allens, Alphachimp, Alterego, Amaltheus, Ammonight423, Andre Engels, Andres, Anna Lincoln, AnnaFrance, Anthere, Antipastor, Ap, ArielGold, Arpingstone, Art LaPella, Artat, Ashmoo, Atakdoug, Atulsnischal, Aua, Avia, Avs5221, Awesomator1, AxelBoldt, Baa, Baby mami 101, Backwalker, BanyanTree, Beetstra, Beland, BengMog, Besidesamiracle, Bgold, Billy55566666, Birdkid100, Blanchardb, Bobblewik, Bobbo, Bobo192, Boccobrock, Boing! said Zebedee, Bookinhand, Bradv, Brendanconway, Brian0918, Brya, Bryan Derksen, Bueller 007, Burner0718, Busaccsb, C.Fred, C8755, CFH7, CRGreathouse, CWii, CYD, Cac070489, Caltas, Can't sleep, clown will eat me, Candorwien, Capricorn42, Captain B, Card, CardinalDan, Catgut, Cfailde, Chill doubt, Choess, Chriss789, Christian75, Chunminghan, Chyeahdawg, Circeus, Citynoise, Cmdrjameson, Conversion script, Crusadeonilliteracy, Curps, Cygnis insignis, D-Notice, Daderot, Daniel5127, Danielgdm, Dave.Dunford, Dawn Bard, Dawright12, Dbachmann, Dead3y3, Dendrid, Denisarona, Devrit, Dmeranda, Dmsdjing, DonMacneill, Doulos Christos, Dover, Dr Oldekop, Dratman, Dreadstar, Dyanega, Dysmorodrepanis, EcoNerd1986, Ed Poor, Ed.howland, Edison, Edonovan, Eddie123, El C, Eleassar, Elekhh, Eliorcohen, Elliskev, EncycloPetey, Enok Walker, Epbr123, ErkDemon, Escape Orbit, Eshstevebaugh, Ettrig, Euchiasmus, Evercat, Everyking, Ezhuttukari, FF2010, FaEu, Fastfission, Fieldday-sunday, Figma, First Light, FlopTopSet, Flowerpotman, Flyguy649, Fordmadoxfraud, FranciscoWelterSchultes, Fredrik, Frozen4322, Fyrael, GTBacchus, Garethball, Gary King, Gdarin, Gdr, GeorgeMoney, GerardM, Giantsshoulders, Giftlite, Gilliam, Ginsengbomb, Glenmin, Glenn, Glump, Gnostrat, Goatasaur, God Emperor, GoingBatty, Goldenhotmail, Golnazfotohabadi, Grafen, Graft, Graminophile, Haidata, HappyCamper, Hardyplants, Hephaestos, Heron, Hersfold, Hmrox, Il MusLiM HyBRiD II, IMNOTAVANDALK9, Icairns, Iliveincanadadry, Imacolt, Immunize, Indon, Inge-Lyubov, Intelligentsium, Inter16, Invertzoo, Iridescent, IronGargoyle, ItsZippy, Ixfd64, J.delanoy, JForget, JV Smithy, JaGa, Jabrona, Jackhynes, Jacoplane, Jamesalbert1234, Jefflayman, Jerry Zhang,

Jerryseinfeld, JetLover, Jethrocapone, Jimfbleak, Jimpscott, Jiy, Jj137, Jmelville17, Jmeppley, Jni, Jnp2109, Joelr31, John KB, John Wilkins, John of Reading, John254, Jorend, Josemanimala, Jplflyer, Jptdrake, Jrockley, Jruderman, Julesd, Jusdafax, KVDP, Kamal11992288, Karada, Karebh, Katalaveno, Katieh5584, Katimawan2005, Khalid Mahmood, Kingdon, KlaudiuMihaila, Koavf, Kranix, Ks0stm, Kungfuadam, Kzollman, L Kensington, Lakers, Lalalalalala, Lawerjax, LeaveSleaves, Lesgles, Levineps, Lexor, Limideen, Lizardcuckoo, LonelyBeacon, Look2See1, M fic, M0rphzone, MPF, Maddie!, Magioladitis, Maky, Malo, Marek69, Marshman, Marsoult, Martarius, Mattisse, Mav, Maxis ftw, Mba123, McGeddon, Mdz, Menchi, Mgiganteus1, Michael C Price, Michael Hardy, Monty845, MrOllie, Mspraveen, Naddy, Nadiatalent, Nagy, Nathan, Nativeborncal, Nepenthes, Neuron132, Neutrality, Nikai, Nikita Borisov, Ninukk, Niqueco, Niteowlneils, Nivix, Noodleman, Np105034, Nsaa, ONEder Boy, Obsidian Soul, Ohnoitsjamie, OldakQuill, Oldekop, Orangemarlin, Orphan Wiki, PPdd, Paalexan, Pascal.Tesson, Patrick, Paul Foxworthy, Pauli133, Peak, Pekayer11, Pelago, Pengo, Peter coxhead, Petiatil, Petter Bøckman, Pgk, Phantomsteve, Phexxa, PhilKnight, Philcha, Philg88, Philip Trueman, PierreAbbat, Pinethicket, Pippu d'Angelo, Pjvpjv, Plumbago, Poison iva, PoisonedQuill, Prkapoorvijay, Prodego, Promethean, Quahog5News, Quindraco, R6MaY89, RDBrown, Rajah, Ram-Man, Redaktor, Redgolpe, Reguiieee, Reo On, Res2216firestar, RexNL, Ricardo Ferreira de Oliveira, Rich Farmbrough, Richard001, Rigel may, Rjwilmsi, RoyBoy, Rror, RyanCross, Ryguasu, Samsara, Sasata, Sax Russell, Scavenger-X, Scetoaux, Schewek, SchfiftyThree, Schnolle, Scoot-Overload, Scrantonian, Seglea, Semorrison, SeoMac, Shanes, Shenme, Shoy, Shyamal, SimonP, Sjö, SkyMachine, Slrubenstein, Sluzzelin, Smelialichu, Snalwibma, Snek01, Snowmanradio, SoLando, Sophie means wisdom, Spaully, Speciate, Speight, Spencer, Spiffy sperry, St. Nerol, Standproud1, Steinsky, Stemonitis, Stephen Gilbert, Stephenb, Steven J. Anderson, Stevenmitchell, Steveprutz, Stfg, Sucro, Sunderland06, Sunshine4921, SuperSpeller22, Surfspeczz, Sylverfysh, Szajd, TFCforever, THEN WHO WAS PHONE?, Ta bu shi da yu, Tannin, Taranet, Tavilis, Taztouzi1, Tbhotch, Technopat, Ted Baenziger, Teles, Telesiphe, Temporaluser, The High Fin Sperm Whale, The Letter J, The Mysterious El Willstro, The Thing That Should Not Be, Thibbs, Tide rolls, TimVickers, Timir2, Timo Honkasalo, Tinymonty, Tmangray, Tobias Hoevekamp, Tom David, Tom Radulovich, Tommy2010, Tompw, Tottingshire, Tpbradbury, Trainra, Trans Arctica, Treisijs, Trumpkinius, TutterMouse, Twas Now, Ucucha, UtherSRG, VI, Vallonio, Vanished User 4517, Victor falk, Vina, Vlmastra, Vsmith, Waggers, Wandytoo, Wangry, Wavelength, We.eter, WeGoAndiamo, Weiner2952, Why Not A Duck, Wiki gezza, Wikiality123, Wikibofh, Wikieditor06, Wikih101, Wikipelli, WilyD, Wing gundam, Wings Upon My Feet, Wisdom89, Wknight94, Woohookitty, Wtmitchell, XJamRastafire, Xook1kai Choa6aur, Yahel Guhan, Yamamoto Ichiro, Yes four, Yidisheryid, Zhafts, Zoologyteacher, Zundark, Саша Стефановић, राम, , 719 anonymous edits

Domain_(biology) *Source*: http://en.wikipedia.org/w/index.php?title=Domain_%28biology%29 *Contributors*: 5 albert square, Alksub, Amorymeltzer, Andre Engels, Andres, Angrysockhop, ArdClose, Bcasterline, Biblbroks, Bjankuloski06en, Brya, CT Cooper, Capricorn42, Chiswick Chap, Cognatus, ColinFine, Crium, DGG, Donald Albury, Dondegroovily, Dozols, Eog1916, Fabartus, Gnostrat, Grendelkhan, Gurch, Habbzz, Hiandbaii, Immunize, Iph, Irregulargalaxies, J.delanoy, JWSchmidt, Jandre3895, Jason.grossman, Jay2332, Jeff G., Josh Grosse, Jrockley, KJS77, Katalaveno, Katimawan2005, Keeves, Khajidha, Killervogel5, Lenticel, Lycurgus, Mad Greg, Markhurd, MelkorDCLXVI, Michael Hardy, N2e, Neutrality, NewEnglandYankee, Nihiltres, Nnemo, Northnomad, NotVeryBright, Nuno Tavares, OlEnglish, PAvdK, Pengo, Philcha, Pmaguire, Ranveig, Repku, Rich Farmbrough, Ringbang, Rjwilmsi, RoyBoy, Saebjorn, Salvor, Scwlong, SkY`, Smith609, Snek01, Sombrus, SpaceFalcon2001, Spidey104, SyntaxError55, Syrthiss, THEN WHO WAS PHONE?, TJSwoboda, Tedder, Tedneeman, The Anome, Tompw, Treisijs, Tresiden, Unyoyega, Victor falk, Vojtech.dostal, Vuong Ngan Ha, Xris0, YoterMimeni, 105 anonymous edits

Juglandaceae *Source*: http://en.wikipedia.org/w/index.php?title=Juglandaceae *Contributors*: Adrian.benko, Askelgwen, Bomac, Borgx, Burhan br, Calliopejen1, Circeus, Donarreiskoffer, EncycloPetey, Erud, Fanghong, Glenn, Griensteidl, Hesperian, Immanuel Giel, Jay L09, Jimfbleak, Jmorgan, Josh Grosse, Kazubon, Kenraiz, Kevmin, Kpjas, MPF, MrDarwin, Muriel Gottrop, Naddy, Nk, Palica, Rjwilmsi, Rkitko, SB Johnny, SilkTork, Slaweks, Sobreira, Stan Shebs, TDogg310, Unyoyega, UtherSRG, Vald, Vuong Ngan Ha, Wiwaxia, Wwm101, 9 anonymous edits

Hickory *Source*: http://en.wikipedia.org/w/index.php?title=Hickory *Contributors*: 12835S, 17Drew, 28421u2232nfenfcenc, Aaron Walden, Abrahami, Academic Challenger, Acalamari, Alansohn, Amcbride, Andy M. Wang, Anomalocaris, Anthony Appleyard, Antonio Lopez, Apuma, Architect7, Auntof6, Baindc, Bart133, Baskaufs, Bfpage, Bob Burkhardt, Bruce Marlin, Brutaldeluxe, Brya, Caltas, Caltrop, Carlossuarez46, Circeus, Curb Chain, D3, DanielCD, Davecrossman, Dbanks2, Djlayton4, DocWatson42, Download, Dysmorodrepanis, ESkog, EncycloPetey, Epbr123, Ewen, Fastifex, Fbazzo, Firsfron, Fledgeling, Flinkly, Fyyer, Ghirlandajo, Gigemag76, Guppy2, Halogenated, Hamamelis, Hamiltondaniel, IceCreamAntisocial, Idontknowme, Jelloman1234, Jonkerz, Josh Parris, Joyous!, Karduelis, Kb3edk, Kevmin, Kingdon, Kmanblue, Kuru, Latka, Leuqarte, Liftarn, MER-C, MPF, Magrinder, Matthewcgirling, Melchoir, Mendaliv, Metanoid, Mike Rosoft, Minesweeper, Miss Madeline, Naddy, Nadiatalent, NewEnglandYankee, Noctibus, Od Mishehu, Peter Karlsen, Phlyaristis, Pinethicket, Pollinator, Remilo, Richard Barlow, Rjwilmsi, Rkitko, Rwhittall, S h i v a (Visnu), Schzmo, Secretlondon, SimonP, Sisterdetestai, Sjakkalle, Sligocki, Sluzzelin, Snowolf, Sten, TDogg310, Tanaats, Tatterfly, Tbc2, TheLongTone, Thumperward, Tls, Tony Fox, TooUnoriginalToCreativelyNameAccount, Tristynu, Vrenator, W4chris, Wertuose, Ytfc23, Zzorse, 164 anonymous edits

Taxonomic_rank *Source*: http://en.wikipedia.org/w/index.php?title=Taxonomic_rank *Contributors*: Andrew Dalby, Andycjp, Anonymous101, Assasin Joe, B222, CapitalR, Cntras, CurtisSwain, Cyberscholar, DFRussia, Dcirovic, Debeo Morium, Dendrid, Dysmorodrepanis, ENeville, Excirial, Forja, Freependulum, Fryed-peach, GTBacchus, Gary King, Gerbrant, Gnostrat, Hairy Dude, Hongsy, Human anatomy, Jauhienij, Jeff kuta, Kaldari, Katach, Killiondude, Kloepfer1, Kupirijo, Kwamikagami, Lavateraguy, Libcub, Look2See1, Lpsickle, M Alan Kazlev, Martlet1215, MattOates, MrKIA11, Nadiatalent, Newone, Nurg, Nwayyir, Olegwiki, Olympic god, Ospalh, Oxymoron83, Pastiness, Peter G Werner, Peter coxhead, Pimlottc, Qarel, RPlunk2853, RekishiEJ, Rich Farmbrough, Rklawton, Rocket000, Rojomoke, SC979, SDS, Samak47, ScottMHoward, Shieber, Smartiger, Smith609, Snek01, Soulkeeper, Squids and Chips, Steven J. Anderson, Stillnotelf, SunCreator, Wheedhee, WikiKherad, Wilson44691, Wisdom89, Wknight94, Wlodzimierz, Woohookitty, Ycl6, 91 anonymous edits

Taxon *Source*: http://en.wikipedia.org/w/index.php?title=Taxon *Contributors*: Anaxial, Andres, Andycjp, Anna Frodesiak, Ascánder, Ballista, Barryap, Bodragon, Brya, Bsadowski1, Cameron Nedland, Chris Dubey, Circeus, Craig Butz, Crazyaboutbio, Crout1, DanielCD, David Shay, Dendrid, Dominus, Dysmorodrepanis, Ellywa, EnSamulili, EncycloPetey, Eog1916, Ernsts, Flammifer, Gdarin, GerardM, Gmaxwell, Grika, Gunnar Mikalsen Kvifte, Hashar, Hghyux, Hiplis, House, Huku-chan, ILike2BeAnonymous, Iainrlamb, Ibbel, Invertzoo, Iph, Ix3tdg, J.delanoy, Jan Pospíšil, JerrySteal, JodoYodo, Joeblakesley, JohnnyNyquist, Josh Grosse, Julesd, Lesgles, MPF, MPerel, Mani1, Marcomendezg, Martarius, Materialscientist, Math Champion, Mav, Menchi, Mgiganteus1, MichaK, Montrealais, Mrevan, Nbarth, Nihiltres, Niteowlneils, Nkon1, NotWith, Perspicacite, Pigottsm, Pit, Pol098, Qllach, Quarty, Saga City, Samoawater, Shyamal, Skarebo, Snek01, Spacemanspif, Sunray, Thingg, Tuxide, Two Engineer, Una Smith, UtherSRG, Vanka5, Wavelength, We.eter, Xanthis, 77 anonymous edits

Biological_classification *Source*: http://en.wikipedia.org/w/index.php?title=Biological_classification *Contributors*: 168..., 172.153.96.xxx, 1984, 2004-12-29T22:45Z, 21655, 5 albert square, Abigail-II, Achowat, Ahoerstemeier, Aksi great, Alansohn, Aldaron, Aleator, Alexei Kouprianov, Alexkin, Aljullu, Allicat07, Allstarecho, Alone Coder, Alpha Quadrant (alt), Ameliorate!, AmiDaniel, Amorymeltzer, Ancheta Wis, Andonic, AndriuZ, AndyCapp, Angr, Animum, Anlace, Anomalocaris, Anomaly2002, Anonymous editor, Antandrus, Antonio Lopez, Apokryltaros, Arendedwinter, Arensb, AshLin, Ashot Gabrielyan, Atif.t2, Aude, AxelBoldt, Bacon and the Sandwich, Baldhur, Ballista, Barkeep, BarretB, Bcasterline, Beano, Because the mail never stops, Beccaa94, Beland, Belg4mit, Bencherlite, Berria, Berton, Betterusername, Billymac00, Biopresto, Blackburn.greg, Blazotron, Blotto adrift, Bobo192, Borislav, Bridesmill, Brockert, BrokenSegue, Brya, Bryan Derksen, BryanG, Bucketsofg, Bugboy52.40, Burner0718, Burntsauce, CJLL Wright, CJTweedy, CWii, Cacao43, Cactus26, Cadaeib, Cadiomals, Calabe1992, Calaschysm, Caltas, Calvin677, Can't sleep, clown will eat me, Canadian Paul, CanisRufus, CapitalR, Capricorn42, CardinalDan, Casliber, Cenarium, Cephal-odd, Chaleyer61, Chilepine, ChongDae, Chorobek, Chun-hian, CiTrusD, Ckampmeier, Clarince63, ClockworkSoul, Closedmouth, Cohee, CohenTheBavarian, Cometstyles, Comm. makatau, Conversion script, Courcelles, Cp420, Cromwellt, Croq, Cureden, Curtis Clark, D, DMacks, DRE, Daft punkette, Dan Koehl, Danarmak, DancingPenguin, Danger, Danielkwalsh, Danilot, Dante Alighieri, David Kernow, David spector, Davodd, Dcattell, DerHexer, Dinoguy2, Dirgela, Discospinster, Disneyfreak96, Dixi, Dlohcierekim, Dmanning, Dobrydneyj, Donald Albury, Donarreiskoffer, Dougweller, Dr.Bastedo, Dragoneye776, DragonflySixtyseven, Dreadstar, Dstar3k, Dwayne, Dyanega, Dysmorodrepanis, E rulez, EWS23, EamonnPKeane, Eastlaw, Edward321, El C, Eleassar, Eliz81, Ellergodt, Emily Jensen, Enviroboy, Eog1916, Epbr123, Eras-mus, Eric Forste, Erkan Yilmaz, Eubulides, Eugene van der Pijll, Everyking, Excirial, Fabartus, Falcon Kirtaran, FeralDruid, Figma, Flewis, Flowerparty, Fluffernutter, Flying Saucer, FreplySpang, Funnyfarmofdoom, Fuzheado, Fæ, GPHemsley, Gaijin42, Gail, Gaius Cornelius, Galoubet, Gandalf1491, Gary King, Gautam p, Gdr, Gearmaster09, Geeoharee, GerardM, Gfoley4, Ghostdood, Giftlite, Gilliam, Glane23, Glenn, Gnostrat, GorillaWarfare, Gracefool, Graham Chapman, Graham87, Granitethighs, Greatal386, Groessler, Grundle2600, Guilee186, Gurch, Gutworth, HJKeats, Hadal, HalJor, Halvard, Hardyplants, Harizotoh9, Hdante, Hectorthebat, Heman, Heron, Hires an editor, Hobartimus, Hodja Nasreddin, Honza Záruba, Hughcharlesparker, Huhsunqu, Hurricane111, Husond, IW.HG, Ian Pitchford, Igiffin, Ilovedulu, IndigoSeptimus, Instinct, Intgr, Into The Fray, Introscop, Invertzoo, Iridescent, Is is Is, Istvan, J. Spencer, J.delanoy, JDspeeder1, Jaknouse, JamesBWatson, Jamesalaska, Jamesofur, Jason.grossman, Jasonandyou, Jauhienij, Jecar, Jerry Zhang, Jh51681, JinJian, Jjmontalbo, Jmeppley, JohnCub, Johnuniq, Joseph Solis in Australia, Josh Grosse, Joymmart, Jpatokal, KNHaw, Karebh, Kartben9, Kathryn NicDhàna, Kbdank71, Keilana, Keith Edkins, Kel-nage, Kemiv, Kevin.cohen, Khalid Mahmood, KimvdLinde, Kingdon, Kku, KnowledgeOfSelf, Koektrommel, Kotniski, Krawi, Krukouski, Kupirijo, KyraVixen, L1I2I3I4I5I6I7I8I9, Landon1980, Lanthanum-138, Laookmen, Larryincinci, Lavateraguy, Leandrod, LeaveSleaves, Leeyc0, Legaleagle86, Lenticel, Leptictidium, Lerdthenerd, Lesgles, Levineps, Lexor, LiDaobing, LibLord, Life of Riley, Lindsay658, Little Mountain 5, LittleOldMe, Livajo, Lmc169, Logan, Looxix, Los deits, Lucyin, Luna Santin, M.nelson, MER-C, MKoltnow, MPF, MSJapan, MagneticFlux, Majvr, Mani1, Manuelt15, Manway, Marek69, MarsRover, Master Jay, Mathonius, Maurreen, Mav, McSly, Mdd, Meelar, Mejor Los Indios, Michael Hardy, Mike Rosoft, Minghong, Miquonranger03, MissAlyx, Miszal3, MithrandirAgain, Moink, Moomoomoo, Morning277, Mowgli, Mr pand, Mr. Lefty, MrDarwin, Mrhobbz, Mrssandman, Mschel, Muntuwandi, Mwng, Mxn, Myrmecos, N3X15, N5iln, NHRHS2010, Nadiatalent, NawlinWiki, Nayvik, NeilN, NeoJustin, Nguyen Thanh Quang, Nick1nildram, Nicolae Coman, Nihiltres, Nivix, Nneonneo, Norwikian, Notafly, NovaDog, Nsaa, Nufy8, Nunh-huh, Nuno Tavares, ONUnicorn, Obsidian Soul, Ocdncntx, Oemb1905, Ojs, Old Father Time, Old Moonraker, OldakQuill, Oliver Pereira, Omodaka, Onco p53, Optakeover, Orange ginger, Otolemur crassicaudatus, Ouzo, PDH, PM800, PatPeter, Paul August, Peak, Pengo, Perfect Proposal, Peter, Peter coxhead, Petru Dimitriu, Petter Bøckman, Phil1988, Philip Trueman, Phyzome, PierreAbbat, Pihka, Pikachuwashere, Pinethicket, Pippu d'Angelo, Poohbear 0226, Postoak, Prashanthns, Princessamoeba, Proofreader77, Pseudomonas, Pym98, Quantpole, Quiddity, RC-0722, RK, Radagast83, Ranveig, Raz1el, Rds1970, Rdsmith4, Red Winged Duck, Reesyo, Regibox, Remember the dot, Renegadeshark, RexNL, Rgamble, Riana, RichardF, Ridnfrk7, Rizniz, Rkitko, Rocastelo, RogerHyam, Roland2, Romanm, Ronbo76, Ronhjones, Rory096, Rossami, RoyBoy, RyanCross, Salvio giuliano, SchfiftyThree, Scholar1975, Scooter4, Scottalter, Seascapeza, SebastianHelm, Seglea, Semperf, Sentausa, Seqsea, Shafei, Shizhao, Shoes101, Sideways713, Sjwk, Sjö, Smith609, Snek01, Snigbrook, Snowmanradio, Snoyes, Snyper666, Special-T, Specs112, SpeedyGonsales, Stemonitis, Stevertigo, Summer Song, SupernovaExplosion, Syp, THE MIST, TUF-KAT, Taco325i, Tannin, Tau'olunga, Tcatron565, Tdslk, TeaDrinker, Tellyaddict, Temporarily Insane, Tgeairn, The Anome, The Rambling Man, The Thing That Should Not Be, TheBlueFlamingo, Thedjatclubrock, Theresa knott, Tiddly Tom, Tide rolls, Tiggerjay, Tim1357, Timc, Timir2, Tiptoety, Tkinias, Tobby72, Todfox, Tom harrison, Tommy2010, Tompw, Tomtom547, Tony Daly, Tpbradbury, Trusilver, Tuganax, Tvdm, Twinkler4, Ubiq, Ulric1313, Ultimateidiot, Uncle Dick, Uppland, Useight, UtherSRG, Vedantm, Vera.tetrix, Versus22, Violask81976, Virek, Viridian, Viriditas, Vsmith, Wasbeer, Wavelength, Wayward, Welsh, WhiteCat, Wickey-nl, Wik, Wikid77, Wikipelli, Wilke, Will Beback Auto, Willtron, Wimt, Wind, Windchaser, Wisdom89, Wknight94, Wlodzimierz, Wulgulmerang, Xionbox, Yelloeyes, Yeom0609, Yosri, Ytrottier, Zariane, Zidonuke, Zigger, Zoicon5, ZyaX, Zzuuzz, `erin`, Гатерас, ТимофейЛееСуда, Шизомби, 1366 anonymous edits

Image Sources, Licenses and Contributors

File:Biological_classification_L_Pengo_vflip.svg *Source*: http://en.wikipedia.org/w/index.php?title=File:Biological_classification_L_Pengo_vflip.svg *License*: unknown *Contributors*: Adrignola, ArnoLagrange, Nisetpdajsankha, Pavel55, Pengo

File:Phylloscopus trochiloides NAUMANN.jpg *Source*: http://en.wikipedia.org/w/index.php?title=File:Phylloscopus_trochiloides_NAUMANN.jpg *License*: unknown *Contributors*: Anniolek, Kilom691, Nicke L, Red devil 666

File:Undiscovered species chart.png *Source*: http://en.wikipedia.org/w/index.php?title=File:Undiscovered_species_chart.png *License*: unknown *Contributors*: User:KVDP

File:Carolus Linnaeus (cleaned up version).jpg *Source*: http://en.wikipedia.org/w/index.php?title=File:Carolus_Linnaeus_(cleaned_up_version).jpg *License*: unknown *Contributors*: Original painting by Alexander Roslin. Digitally improved by Greg L.

file:Juglans regia Broadview.jpg *Source*: http://en.wikipedia.org/w/index.php?title=File:Juglans_regia_Broadview.jpg *License*: unknown *Contributors*: Common Good, Rasbak

File:Red Pencil Icon.png *Source*: http://en.wikipedia.org/w/index.php?title=File:Red_Pencil_Icon.png *License*: unknown *Contributors*: User:Peter coxhead

Image:Walnut03.jpg *Source*: http://en.wikipedia.org/w/index.php?title=File:Walnut03.jpg *License*: unknown *Contributors*: Fir0002, Skipjack, Wst, 1 anonymous edits

Image:Platycarya strobilacea1.jpg *Source*: http://en.wikipedia.org/w/index.php?title=File:Platycarya_strobilacea1.jpg *License*: unknown *Contributors*:

file:Carya Morton 29-U-10.jpg *Source*: http://en.wikipedia.org/w/index.php?title=File:Carya_Morton_29-U-10.jpg *License*: unknown *Contributors*: User:Bruce Marlin

File:Carya cordiformis.jpg *Source*: http://en.wikipedia.org/w/index.php?title=File:Carya_cordiformis.jpg *License*: unknown *Contributors*: User:MPF

File:Hickory nuts 6060.JPG *Source*: http://en.wikipedia.org/w/index.php?title=File:Hickory_nuts_6060.JPG *License*: unknown *Contributors*: Abrahami, MPF, TeunSpaans

File:Carya nuts.jpg *Source*: http://en.wikipedia.org/w/index.php?title=File:Carya_nuts.jpg *License*: unknown *Contributors*: User:Melchoir

image:Elephants in Kenya.jpg *Source*: http://en.wikipedia.org/w/index.php?title=File:Elephants_in_Kenya.jpg *License*: unknown *Contributors*: User:Sa-se

File:Aristotle Altemps Inv8575.jpg *Source*: http://en.wikipedia.org/w/index.php?title=File:Aristotle_Altemps_Inv8575.jpg *License*: unknown *Contributors*: User:Jastrow

Image:Rhinoceros in Gesner's 1551 Historiae animalium.jpg *Source*: http://en.wikipedia.org/w/index.php?title=File:Rhinoceros_in_Gesner's_1551_Historiae_animalium.jpg *License*: unknown *Contributors*: Conrad Gesner

File:Carl von Linné2.jpg *Source*: http://en.wikipedia.org/w/index.php?title=File:Carl_von_Linné2.jpg *License*: unknown *Contributors*: Kaganer, Limulus, Materialscientist, Shakko

File:Spindle diagram.jpg *Source*: http://en.wikipedia.org/w/index.php?title=File:Spindle_diagram.jpg *License*: unknown *Contributors*: User:Petter Bøckman

File:Cladogram vertebrata.jpg *Source*: http://en.wikipedia.org/w/index.php?title=File:Cladogram_vertebrata.jpg *License*: unknown *Contributors*: User:Petter Bøckman

GNU Free Documentation License Version 1.2, November 2002 Copyright (C) 2000,2001,2002 Free Software Foundation, Inc. 59 Temple Place, Suite 330, Boston, MA 02111-1307 USA Everyone is permitted to copy and distribute verbatim copies of this license document, but changing it is not allowed.

0. PREAMBLE

The purpose of this License is to make a manual, textbook, or other functional and useful document "free" in the sense of freedom: to assure everyone the effective freedom to copy and redistribute it, with or without modifying it, either commercially or noncommercially. Secondarily, this License preserves for the author and publisher a way to get credit for their work, while not being considered responsible for modifications made by others. This License is a kind of "copyleft", which means that derivative works of the document must themselves be free in the same sense. It complements the GNU General Public License, which is a copyleft license designed for free software. We have designed this License in order to use it for manuals for free software, because free software needs free documentation: a free program should come with manuals providing the same freedoms that the software does. But this License is not limited to software manuals; it can be used for any textual work, regardless of subject matter or whether it is published as a printed book. We recommend this License principally for works whose purpose is instruction or reference.

1. APPLICABILITY AND DEFINITIONS

This License applies to any manual or other work, in any medium, that contains a notice placed by the copyright holder saying it can be distributed under the terms of this License. Such a notice grants a world-wide, royalty-free license, unlimited in duration, to use that work under the conditions stated herein. The "Document", below, refers to any such manual or work. Any member of the public is a licensee, and is addressed as "you". You accept the license if you copy, modify or distribute the work in a way requiring permission under copyright law. A "Modified Version" of the Document means any work containing the Document or a portion of it, either copied verbatim, or with modifications and/or translated into another language. A "Secondary Section" is a named appendix or a front-matter section of the Document that deals exclusively with the relationship of the publishers or authors of the Document to the Document's overall subject (or to related matters) and contains nothing that could fall directly within that overall subject. (Thus, if the Document is in part a textbook of mathematics, a Secondary Section may not explain any mathematics.) The relationship could be a matter of historical connection with the subject or with related matters, or of legal, commercial, philosophical, ethical or political position regarding them. The "Invariant Sections" are certain Secondary Sections whose titles are designated, as being those of Invariant Sections, in the notice that says that the Document is released under this License. If a section does not fit the above definition of Secondary then it is not allowed to be designated as Invariant. The Document may contain zero Invariant Sections. If the Document does not identify any Invariant Sections then there are none. The "Cover Texts" are certain short passages of text that are listed, as Front-Cover Texts or Back-Cover Texts, in the notice that says that the Document is released under this License. A Front-Cover Text may be at most 5 words, and a Back-Cover Text may be at most 25 words. A "Transparent" copy of the Document means a machine-readable copy, represented in a format whose specification is available to the general public, that is suitable for revising the document straightforwardly with generic text editors or (for images composed of pixels) generic paint programs or (for drawings) some widely available drawing editor, and that is suitable for input to text formatters or for automatic translation to a variety of formats suitable for input to text formatters. A copy made in an otherwise Transparent file format whose markup, or absence of markup, has been arranged to thwart or discourage subsequent modification by readers is not Transparent. An image format is not Transparent if used for any substantial amount of text. A copy that is not "Transparent" is called "Opaque". Examples of suitable formats for Transparent copies include plain ASCII without markup, Texinfo input format, LaTeX input format, SGML or XML using a publicly available DTD, and standard-conforming simple HTML, PostScript or PDF designed for human modification. Examples of transparent image formats include PNG, XCF and JPG. Opaque formats include proprietary formats that can be read and edited only by proprietary word processors, SGML or XML for which the DTD and/or processing tools are not generally available, and the machine-generated HTML, PostScript or PDF produced by some word processors for output purposes only. The "Title Page" means, for a printed book, the title page itself, plus such following pages as are needed to hold, legibly, the material this License requires to appear in the title page. For works in formats which do not have any title page as such, "Title Page" means the text near the most prominent appearance of the work's title, preceding the beginning of the body of the text. A section "Entitled XYZ" means a named subunit of the Document whose title either is precisely XYZ or contains XYZ in parentheses following text that translates XYZ in another language. (Here XYZ stands for a specific section name mentioned below, such as "Acknowledgements", "Dedications", "Endorsements", or "History".) To "Preserve the Title" of such a section when you modify the Document means that it remains a section "Entitled XYZ" according to this definition. The Document may include Warranty Disclaimers next to the notice which states that this License applies to the Document. These Warranty Disclaimers are considered to be included by reference in this License, but only as regards disclaiming warranties: any other implication that these Warranty Disclaimers may have is void and has no effect on the meaning of this License.

2. VERBATIM COPYING

You may copy and distribute the Document in any medium, either commercially or noncommercially, provided that this License, the copyright notices, and the license notice saying this License applies to the Document are reproduced in all copies, and that you add no other conditions whatsoever to those of this License. You may not use technical measures to obstruct or control the reading or further copying of the copies you make or distribute. However, you may accept compensation in exchange for copies. If you distribute a large enough number of copies you must also follow the conditions in section 3. You may also lend copies, under the same conditions stated above, and you may publicly display copies.

3. COPYING IN QUANTITY

If you publish printed copies (or copies in media that commonly have printed covers) of the Document, numbering more than 100, and the Document's license notice requires Cover Texts, you must enclose the copies in covers that carry, clearly and legibly, all these Cover Texts: Front-Cover Texts on the front cover, and Back-Cover Texts on the back cover. Both covers must also clearly and legibly identify you as the publisher of these copies. The front cover must present the full title with all words of the title equally prominent and visible. You may add other material on the covers in addition. Copying with changes limited to the covers, as long as they preserve the title of the Document and satisfy these conditions, can be treated as verbatim copying in other respects. If the required texts for either cover are too voluminous to fit legibly, you should put the first ones listed (as many as fit reasonably) on the actual cover, and continue the rest onto adjacent pages. If you publish or distribute Opaque copies of the Document numbering more than 100, you must either include a machine-readable Transparent copy along with each Opaque copy, or state in or with each Opaque copy a computer-network location from which the general network-using public has access to download using public-standard network protocols a complete Transparent copy of the Document, free of added material. If you use the latter option, you must take reasonably prudent steps, when you begin distribution of Opaque copies in quantity, to ensure that this Transparent copy will remain thus accessible at the stated location until at least one year after the last time you distribute an Opaque copy (directly or through your agents or retailers) of that edition to the public. It is requested, but not required, that you contact the authors of the Document well before redistributing any large number of copies, to give them a chance to provide you with an updated version of the Document.

4. MODIFICATIONS

You may copy and distribute a Modified Version of the Document under the conditions of sections 2 and 3 above, provided that you release the Modified Version under precisely this License, with the Modified Version filling the role of the Document, thus licensing distribution and modification of the Modified Version to whoever possesses a copy of it. In addition, you must do these things in the Modified Version: A. Use in the Title Page (and on the covers, if any) a title distinct from that of the Document, and from those of previous versions (which should, if there were any, be listed in the History section of the Document). You may use the same title as a previous version if the original publisher of that version gives permission. B. List on the Title Page, as authors, one or more persons or entities responsible for authorship of the modifications in the Modified Version, together with at least five of the principal authors of the Document (all of its principal authors, if it has fewer than five), unless they release you from this requirement. C. State on the Title page the name of the publisher of the Modified Version, as the publisher. D. Preserve all the copyright notices of the Document. E. Add an appropriate copyright notice for your modifications adjacent to the other copyright notices. F. Include, immediately after the copyright notices, a license notice giving the public permission to use the Modified Version under the terms of this License, in the form shown in the Addendum below. G. Preserve in that license notice the full lists of Invariant Sections and required Cover Texts given in the Document's license notice. H. Include an unaltered copy of this License. I. Preserve the section Entitled "History", Preserve its Title, and add to it an item stating at least the title, year, new authors, and publisher of the Modified Version as given on the Title Page. If there is no section Entitled "History" in the Document, create one stating the title, year, authors, and publisher of the Document as given on its Title Page, then add an item describing the Modified Version as stated in the previous sentence. J. Preserve the network location, if any, given in the Document for public access to a Transparent copy of the Document, and likewise the network locations given in the Document for previous versions it was based on. These may be placed in the "History" section. You may omit a network location for a work that was published at least four years before the Document itself, or if the original publisher of the version it refers to gives permission. K. For any section Entitled "Acknowledgements" or "Dedications", Preserve the Title of the section, and preserve in the section all the substance and tone of each of the contributor acknowledgements and/or dedications given therein. L. Preserve all the Invariant Sections of the Document, unaltered in their text and in their titles. Section numbers or the equivalent are not considered part of the section titles. M. Delete any section Entitled "Endorsements". Such a section may not be included in the Modified Version. N. Do not retitle any existing section to be Entitled "Endorsements" or to conflict in title with any Invariant Section. O. Preserve any Warranty Disclaimers. If the Modified Version includes new front-matter sections or appendices that qualify as Secondary Sections and contain no material copied from the Document, you may at your option designate some or all of these sections as invariant. To do this, add their titles to the list of Invariant Sections in the Modified Version's license notice. These titles must be distinct from any other section titles. You may add a section Entitled "Endorsements", provided it contains nothing but endorsements of your Modified Version by various parties--for example, statements of peer review or that the text has been approved by an organization as the authoritative definition of a standard. You may add a passage of up to five words as a Front-Cover Text, and a passage of up to 25 words as a Back-Cover Text, to the end of the list of Cover Texts in the Modified Version. Only one passage of Front-Cover Text and one of Back-Cover Text may be added by (or through arrangements made by) any one entity. If the Document already includes a cover text for the same cover, previously added by you or by arrangement made by the same entity you are acting on behalf of, you may not add another; but you may replace the old one, on explicit permission from the previous publisher that added the old one. The author(s) and publisher(s) of the Document do not by this License give permission to use their names for publicity for or to assert or imply endorsement of any Modified Version.

5. COMBINING DOCUMENTS

You may combine the Document with other documents released under this License, under the terms defined in section 4 above for modified versions, provided that you include in the combination all of the Invariant Sections of all of the original documents, unmodified, and list them all as Invariant Sections of your combined work in its license notice, and that you preserve all their Warranty Disclaimers. The combined work need only contain one copy of this License, and multiple identical Invariant Sections may be replaced with a single copy. If there are multiple Invariant Sections with the same name but different contents, make the title of each such section unique by adding at the end of it, in parentheses, the name of the original author or publisher of that section if known, or else a unique number. Make the same adjustment to the section titles in the list of Invariant Sections in the license notice of the combined work. In the combination, you must combine any sections Entitled "History" in the various original documents, forming one section Entitled "History"; likewise combine any sections Entitled "Acknowledgements", and any sections Entitled "Dedications". You must delete all sections Entitled "Endorsements".

6. COLLECTIONS OF DOCUMENTS

You may make a collection consisting of the Document and other documents released under this License, and replace the individual copies of this License in the various documents with a single copy that is included in the collection, provided that you follow the rules of this License for verbatim copying of each of the documents in all other respects. You may extract a single document from such a collection, and distribute it individually under this License, provided you insert a copy of this License into the extracted document, and follow this License in all other respects regarding verbatim copying of that document.

7. AGGREGATION WITH INDEPENDENT WORKS

A compilation of the Document or its derivatives with other separate and independent documents or works, in or on a volume of a storage or distribution medium, is called an "aggregate" if the copyright resulting from the compilation is not used to limit the legal rights of the compilation's users beyond what the individual works permit. When the Document is included in an aggregate, this License does not apply to the other works in the aggregate which are not themselves derivative works of the Document. If the Cover Text requirement of section 3 is applicable to these copies of the Document, then if the Document is less than one half of the entire aggregate, the Document's Cover Texts may be placed on covers that bracket the Document within the aggregate, or the electronic equivalent of covers if the Document is in electronic form. Otherwise they must appear on printed covers that bracket the whole aggregate.

8. TRANSLATION

Translation is considered a kind of modification, so you may distribute translations of the Document under the terms of section 4. Replacing Invariant Sections with translations requires special permission from their copyright holders, but you may include translations of some or all Invariant Sections in addition to the original versions of these Invariant Sections. You may include a translation of this License, and all the license notices in the Document, and any Warranty Disclaimers, provided that you also include the original English version of this License and the original versions of those notices and disclaimers. In case of a disagreement between the translation and the original version of this License or a notice or disclaimer, the original version will prevail. If a section in the Document is Entitled "Acknowledgements", "Dedications", or "History", the requirement (section 4) to Preserve its Title (section 1) will typically require changing the actual title.

9. TERMINATION

You may not copy, modify, sublicense, or distribute the Document except as expressly provided for under this License. Any other attempt to copy, modify, sublicense or distribute the Document is void, and will automatically terminate your rights under this License. However, parties who have received copies, or rights, from you under this License will not have their licenses terminated so long as such parties remain in full compliance.

10. FUTURE REVISIONS OF THIS LICENSE

The Free Software Foundation may publish new, revised versions of the GNU Free Documentation License from time to time. Such new versions will be similar in spirit to the present version, but may differ in detail to address new problems or concerns. See http://www.gnu.org/copyleft/. Each version of the License is given a distinguishing version number. If the Document specifies that a particular numbered version of this License "or any later version" applies to it, you have the option of following the terms and conditions either of that specified version or of any later version that has been published (not as a draft) by the Free Software Foundation. If the Document does not specify a version number of this License, you may choose any version ever published (not as a draft) by the Free Software Foundation. ADDENDUM: How to use this License for your documents To use this License in a document you have written, include a copy of the License in the document and put the following copyright and license notices just after the title page: Copyright (c) YEAR YOUR NAME. Permission is granted to copy, distribute and/or modify this document under the terms of the GNU Free Documentation License, Version 1.2 or any later version published by the Free Software Foundation; with no Invariant Sections, no Front-Cover Texts, and no Back-Cover Texts. A copy of the license is included in the section entitled "GNU Free Documentation License". If you have Invariant Sections, Front-Cover Texts and Back-Cover Texts, replace the "with...Texts." line with this: with the Invariant Sections being LIST THEIR TITLES, with the Front-Cover Texts being LIST, and with the Back-Cover Texts being LIST. If you have Invariant Sections without Cover Texts, or some other combination of the three, merge those two alternatives to suit the situation. If your document contains nontrivial examples of program code, we recommend releasing these examples in parallel under your choice of free software license, such as the GNU General Public License, to permit their use in free software.

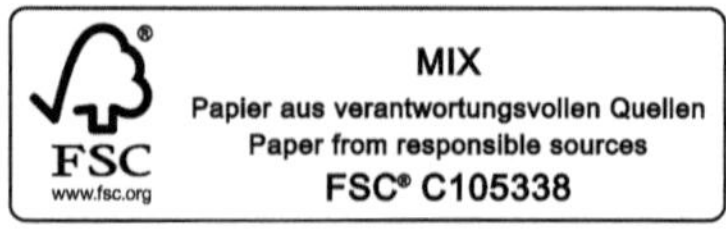

Printed by Books on Demand GmbH, Norderstedt / Germany